Notes on Medical Virology

For Churchill Livingstone

Commissioning Editor Timothy Horne
Project Manager Ninette Premdas
Project Controller Nancy Arnott
Copy Editor Alison Gale
Designer Erik Bigland

Notes on Medical Virology

Morag C. Timbury

MD PhD FRCP (Lon and Glas) FRCPath FRSE
Formerly Director, Central Public Health Laboratory,
Public Health Laboratory Service, Colindale, London

ELEVENTH EDITION

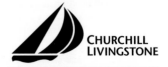

CHURCHILL
LIVINGSTONE

NEW YORK EDINBURGH LONDON MADRID MELBOURNE SAN FRANCISCO AND TOKYO 1997

CHURCHILL LIVINGSTONE
Medical Division of Pearson Professional Limited

Distributed in the United States of America by Churchill
Livingstone Inc., 650 Avenue of the Americas, New York, N.Y.
10011, and by associated companies, branches and
representatives throughout the world.

First published 1967
Eleventh edition 1997   1002091040

Standard edition ISBN 0 443 058458
International edition ISBN 0443 058466

British Library of Cataloguing in Publication Data
A catalogue record for this book is available from the British Library

Library of Congress Cataloging in Publication Data
A catalog record for this book is available from the Library of Congress.

Produced by Longman Asia Ltd, Hong Kong
GCC/01

Medical knowledge is constantly changing. As new information becomes available,
changes in treatment, procedures, equipment and the use of drugs become
necessary. The author and the publishers have, as far as it is possible, taken care to
ensure that the information given in this text is accurate and up to date. However,
readers are strongly advised to confirm that the information, especially with regard
to drug usage, complies with current legislation and standards of practice.

The
publisher's
policy is to use
paper manufactured
from sustainable forests

108322

Preface

This book originated from lecture notes which were handed out to accompany my virology lectures to the medical students while I was Professor of Bacteriology in Glasgow University. I wrote it in the same concise note form to try to present clearly the facts about virus diseases which students need to know for their professional examinations in microbiology. Medical virology has changed with the introduction of molecular technology and for this 11th edition the book has been extensively revised. Although it is meant to be reasonably comprehensive, students should refer to some of the larger books on the subject and I have listed some of my favourites on page 187.

Many colleagues have helped me through advice and discussion, and I am especially grateful to Dr Philip Mortimer of the Virus Reference Division of the Central Public Health Laboratory, Colindale, London, for his help with this edition. I should like to thank colleagues who went to considerable trouble to supply me with the excellent electron micrographs and the colour photographs which show some of the interesting diseases that viruses cause – for the photographs I owe a particular debt of gratitude to Dr A K Chaudhuri, of the Department of Infectious Diseases, Monklands Hospital, Airdrie. Thanks are due to Mr John Gibson of the Department of Medical Illustration of the Central Public Health Laboratory for his advice and help with the illustrations, and to Mr R Callander, who prepared the drawings and diagrams. I shall always be grateful to Professor J H Subak-Sharpe for the many formative and enjoyable years I spent in his department, and to Professor N R Grist in whose laboratory I first acquired my interest in viruses. Finally, I want to thank the editorial staff of Churchill Livingstone for the happy collaboration I have enjoyed with them over nearly 30 years.

London 1997   M.C.T.

Contents

1. Viruses, general properties, disease and host response   1
2. Virus replication   13
3. Laboratory diagnosis of virus infection   27
4. Influenza   37
5. Other respiratory tract infections   45
6. Neurological diseases due to viruses   55
7. Enterovirus infections   59
8. Viral gastroenteritis   67
9. Arthropod-borne virus infections   73
10. Rabies, non-arthropod-borne haemorrhagic fevers   81
11. Herpesvirus diseases   93
12. Childhood fevers   111
13. Poxvirus diseases   123
14. Viral hepatitis   127
15. Chronic neurological diseases due to viruses   141
16. Warts   149
17. Retroviruses   153
18. Antiviral therapy   165
19. Chlamydial diseases   171
20. Rickettsial diseases   177
21. Mycoplasma   183
      Recommended reading   187
      Index   189

1. Viruses, general properties, disease and host response

Viruses are the smallest known infective agents. Most forms of life – animals, plants and bacteria – are susceptible to infection with appropriate viruses.

Three main properties distinguish viruses from other micro-organisms:

1. *Small size*: viruses are smaller than other organisms, although they vary considerably in size – from 10 nm to 300 nm. In contrast, bacteria are approximately 1000 nm and erythrocytes are 7500 nm in diameter.

2. *Genome*: the genome of viruses may be either DNA or RNA; viruses contain only one kind of nucleic acid.

3. *Metabolically inert*: viruses have no metabolic activity outside susceptible host cells. They do not possess active ribosomes or protein-synthesizing apparatus although some viruses contain enzymes within their particles.

Viruses, therefore, can multiply only inside living cells, not on inanimate media. Inside a susceptible cell, the virus redirects the cell's synthesizing machinery to the manufacture of new virus components. It does this by transcription of the virus genome or nucleic acid into virus-specific messenger or mRNA (sometimes the incoming genome can act as this), which then directs the cell to the replication of new virus particles.

VIRUS STRUCTURE

Viruses consist basically of a core of nucleic acid – the *genome* – surrounded by a protein coat. The protein coat protects the viral genome from inactivation by adverse environmental factors, e.g. nucleases in the bloodstream. It is antigenic and often responsible for stimulating the production of protective antibodies.

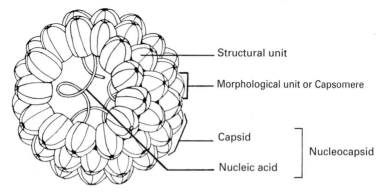

Fig. 1.1   Icosahedral virus particle with cubic symmetry. (Reproduced, with permission, from Madeley C R Virus morphology.)

The *structures* which make up a virus particle are known as:

- **Virion**: the intact virus particle
- **Capsid**: the protein coat
- **Capsomeres**: the protein structural units of which the capsid is composed
- **Nucleic acid genome**: either DNA or RNA
- **Envelope**: the particles of many viruses are surrounded by a lipoprotein envelope, containing viral antigens but also partly derived from the outer membrane or, in some cases, the nuclear membrane of the host cell.

Virus particles show three types of *symmetry*:

1. **Cubic**: in which the particle is an icosahedral protein shell with the nucleic acid contained inside (Fig. 1.1).
2. **Helical**: in which the particle contains an elongated *nucleocapsid*; the capsomeres are arranged round the spiral of nucleic acid (Fig. 1.2). Most helical viruses possess an outer envelope, which invests the helical nucleoprotein.
3. **Complex**: in which the particle does not conform to either cubic or helical symmetry.

CULTIVATION OF VIRUSES

Since viruses can only replicate within living cells, special methods have to be employed for culture in vitro. Three main systems are used for their cultivation in the laboratory (see also Ch. 3):

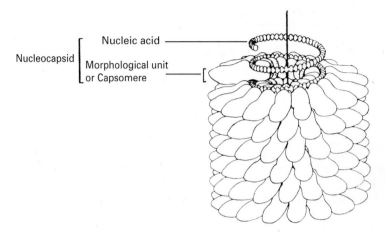

Fig. 1.2   Nucleocapsid of virus particle with helical symmetry. (Reproduced, with permission, from Advances in Virus Research 1960, p. 274.)

1. **Tissue culture**: cells obtained from humans or animals grown in artificial culture in glass vessels in the laboratory: the cells are living and metabolizing and so can support viral replication.

2. **Chick embryo**: some viruses grow in the cells of the chick embryo: now largely superseded by tissue culture, but still used for the preparation of some viral vaccines.

3. **Laboratory animals**: before other techniques were available, viruses were isolated and studied mainly by inoculation of laboratory animals such as mice, rabbits, ferrets and monkeys; animals are still required for the isolation of a few viruses.

EFFECTS OF VIRUSES ON CELLS

Viruses may affect cells in four ways:

1. **Death**: the infection is lethal: it causes a cytopathic effect (CPE) which kills the cell.

2. **Transformation**: the cell is not killed, but is changed from a normal cell to one with the properties of a malignant or cancerous cell.

3. **Latent infection**: the virus remains within the cell in a potentially active state, but produces no obvious effects on the cell's functions.

Table 1.1   Classification of DNA viruses and their diseases

Family	Viruses	Diseases
Poxviruses	variola	smallpox
	molluscum	molluscum contagiosum
Herpesviruses	herpes simplex	herpes
	varicella-zoster	chickenpox, shingles
	cytomegalovirus	infection in the immunocompromised
	EB (Epstein-Barr) virus	infectious mononucleosis
	HHV 6	exanthema subitum
Adenoviruses	adenoviruses	sore throat, conjunctivitis
Hepadnaviruses	hepatitis B	hepatitis
Papovaviruses	papilloma	warts
	JC virus	progressive multifocal leucoencephalopathy
Parvoviruses	B19	erythema infectiosum, aplastic crises

4. *Haemadsorption*: some viruses have protein (haemag-glutinin) in their outer coats, which adheres to erythrocytes causing them to agglutinate: in tissue culture, these viruses produce haemagglutinin on the surface of infected cells, to which added erythrocytes adhere.

CLASSIFICATION

Viruses are assigned to *groups*, mainly on the basis of the morphology of the virus particle, but also of their nucleic acid and method of RNA transcription.

A simplified scheme of classification of the main groups of medically important viruses and the diseases they cause is shown in Tables 1.1 and 1.2. (*Note*: virus families are now known by Latin names. The more widely used anglicized names are used in this classification and throughout the text.)

Diagrams of some representative virus particles are shown in Figure 1.3.

Table 1.2 Classification of RNA viruses and their diseases

Family	Viruses	Diseases
Orthomyxoviruses	influenza	influenza
Paramyxoviruses	parainfluenza respiratory syncytial }	respiratory infection
	measles	measles
	mumps	mumps
Coronaviruses	coronavirus	respiratory infection
Rhabdoviruses	rabies	rabies
Picornaviruses	enteroviruses	meningitis, paralysis
	rhinoviruses	colds
	hepatitis A	hepatitis
Caliciviruses	SRSVs (small round structured viruses)	gastroenteritis
Togaviruses	alphaviruses (Group A arboviruses)	encephalitis, haemorrhagic fevers
	rubivirus	rubella
Flaviviruses	flaviviruses (Group B arboviruses)	encephalitis, haemorrhagic fevers
	hepatitis C	hepatitis
Bunyaviruses	some arboviruses	encephalitis, haemorrhagic fevers
	hantavirus	fever, renal involvement
Reoviruses	rotavirus	gastroenteritis
Arenaviruses	lymphocytic choriomeningitis	meningitis
	Machupo virus Junin virus Lassa virus }	haemorrhagic fevers
Retroviruses	HTLV-I, II	T cell leukaemia, lymphoma, paresis
	HIV-1, 2	AIDS
Filoviruses	Marburg virus	Marburg disease
	Ebola virus	Ebola haemorrhagic fever

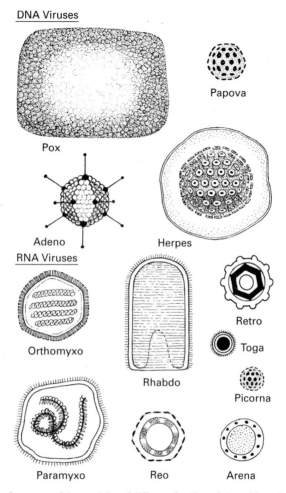

Fig. 1.3   Structure of the particles of different families of virus. *Note*: these drawings are schematic and are not drawn to scale, although differences in relative size are indicated.

The Effect of Physical and Chemical Agents on Viruses

- *Heat*: most are inactivated at 56°C for 30 min or at 100°C for a few seconds.
- *Cold*: stable at low temperatures, most can be stored satisfactorily at −70°C. Some viruses are partially inactivated by the process of freezing and thawing.

- *Drying*: variable: some survive well, others are rapidly inactivated.
- *Ultraviolet irradiation*: inactivates viruses.
- *Chloroform, ether and other organic solvents*: viruses with lipid-containing envelopes are inactivated; those without envelopes are resistant.
- *Oxidizing and reducing agents*: viruses are inactivated by formaldehyde, chlorine, iodine and hydrogen peroxide.
- *β-propiolactone and formaldehyde*: are used for inactivation of viruses for vaccine preparation.
- *Phenols*: most viruses are relatively resistant.
- *Virus disinfectants*: the best are hypochlorite solution (which is corrosive) and glutaraldehyde (which can cause sensitization and irritation to users).

VIRUS DISEASES

Viruses are important and common causes of human disease, especially in children. Most viral infections are mild and the patient makes a complete recovery; many are silent in that the virus multiplies in the body without causing any symptoms at all. However, viral infections which are usually mild sometimes cause severe disease in an unusually susceptible patient. A few viral diseases are severe and always have a high mortality rate.

Entry

Viruses enter the body in four main ways:

1. *Inhalation*: via the respiratory tract
2. *Ingestion*: via the gastrointestinal tract
3. *Inoculation*: through skin abrasions; mucous membranes (e.g. sexual transmission); transfusion; injections (e.g. by doctors or via shared syringes in drug abuse); transplants; via the bite of an arthropod or other animal
4. *Congenital*: i.e. from mother to fetus.

Invasiveness

The main pathogenic mechanism of viruses is invasion. Disease is produced by the direct spread of viruses to tissues and organs. Virus replication in cells usually – although not always – kills the infected cells. This cytopathic effect in vivo causes lesions and so dysfunction in the tissue or organ concerned, with associated symptoms and signs.

Note: in some virus infections, the immune response contributes to the pathogenesis of virus lesions.

HOST RESPONSE TO VIRUS INFECTION

The body's defence mechanisms to virus infection are of two types:

1. Nonspecific
2. Specific.

Nonspecific defence mechanisms

The body has defences which are not specifically directed at particular infectious agents, but which serve as non-immunological barriers to infection:

1. ***Skin***: an effective and impermeable barrier unless breached by injury, disease, etc.

2. ***Respiratory tract***: upward flow of mucus by ciliated epithelium removes virus particles, to prevent invasion of the lower respiratory tract.

3. ***Gastrointestinal tract***: stomach acid inactivates acid-labile viruses. Bile (which lyses enveloped viruses), movement of intestinal contents and uptake of virus by lymphoid tissue all aid elimination of ingested viruses.

4. ***Urinary tract***: flow of urine exerts a protective flushing effect.

5. ***Conjunctiva***: tears flush viruses from the eye.

6. ***Phagocytosis***: an important defence mechanism in bacterial infection and in virus infections also: invading viruses – like bacteria – are ingested by two types of scavenger cell:
    (a) *neutrophil polymorphonuclear leucocytes*
    (b) *macrophages* (or mononuclear cells of the reticuloendothelial system) – of two types:
        (i) free macrophages in lung alveoli, peritoneum
        (ii) fixed macrophages in lymph nodes, spleen, liver (Kupffer cells), connective tissue (histiocytes) and CNS (microglia).

Phagocytosis is enhanced by antibody (a specific immune mechanism) and complement: this effect is known as *opsonization*.

Macrophages 'activated' by cytokines released by T lymphocytes (a specific immune mechanism) have increased phagocytic activity, and are attracted by chemotaxis to the site of infection.

Specific (immunological) defence mechanisms

Immunological responses are of two types:

1. *Humoral* – main effect is neutralization of viruses: responsible for protective immunity
2. *Cellular* – main effect is localization of lesions: kills virus-infected cells.

This complex of immunological reactions is the major body defence, which localizes and eliminates the acute virus infection, the response being directed towards the destruction of virus-infected cells. Clearly antibody has a role in the cellular response and also aids the elimination of virus directly, through its specific and effective neutralizing activity.

Humoral (antibody) response

Like other infectious agents, viruses induce production of antibodies in the blood. Antibodies are:

1. *Immunoglobulins*: proteins which react specifically with antigens – which are also usually proteins, and of which the most important in protective immunity are those on the surface of virus particles.
2. *Produced by plasma cells*: formed when B lymphocytes are activated by encounter with antigen. B lymphocytes have immunoglobulin on their surface, which acts as receptor for virus antigen. Helper T cells contribute to the differentiation of B cells into plasma cells.
3. *Y-shaped*: the stem is the Fc fragment, which activates complement and binds to receptors on infected host cells: the two arms are the Fab fragments and contain the antibody-combining sites.

Three immunoglobulins are mainly responsible for humoral immunity in virus infections:

1. *IgM*: the earliest antibody produced: appears at a variable interval after exposure, depending on the virus, incubation period, dose and route of transmission; persists for about 4–6 weeks, sometimes longer; a pentamer of five IgG molecules.

2. *IgG*: formed later than IgM but persists long term, often for years: responsible for immunity to reinfection.

3. *IgA*: a dimeric molecule, found in body secretions (as well as blood), i.e. saliva, respiratory secretions, tears and intestinal contents; the main antibody involved in immunity to respiratory viruses and in gut immunity associated with enteric virus infection; secretory IgA acquires a carbohydrate 'transport piece' in extracellular fluids that is absent from serum IgA.

Antiviral effects of antibodies:

1. *Neutralization*: antiviral antibodies neutralize virus infectivity and are the principal mechanism for the immunity – often lifelong – which follows virus infection and prevents reinfection.

2. *Antibody-dependent cell-mediated cytotoxicity* (see below).

Cell-mediated immunity

Cellular immunity plays an important part in the response of the body to viruses. For example, children with congenital deficiency of cellular immunity are abnormally susceptible to virus infection and often (although not always) develop unusually severe disease: those with humoral immune deficiency, on the other hand, respond normally to virus infections. Cell-mediated immunity is the mechanism for the elimination of virus-infected cells – and therefore virus – from the body. T or thymus-dependent lymphocytes are the principal cells involved in this. There are two main types:

1. *CD4-positive helper Tcells*: carry CD4 receptors as markers on their surface. The most important cells in the cellular response, they liberate *cytokines* (see below) that activate and modulate cellular immune responses. They require MHC (Major Histocompatibility Complex) Class II antigens to be presented in association with the target antigen for their activation. They also interact with B lymphocytes for antibody production.

2. *CD8-positive cytotoxic T cells*: carry the marker CD8 receptor on their surface and are MHC Class I antigen-restricted. They lyse target cells such as virus-infected cells and tumour cells; the main mechanism for elimination of virus-infected cells from the body; also release cytokines.

Suppressor function: note that both CD4 and CD8 cells can suppress as well as activate the cellular response.

Virus is recognized as antigen by helper T cells when presented by a macrophage or dendritic cell (found in lymph nodes and skin) acting as an antigen-presenting cell: recognition is dependent on MHC Class II antigens.

Lysis of virus-infected cells is mediated by several mechanisms:

1. **Non-antibody-dependent cytotoxicity**: is mediated by three types of lymphocyte:
   (a) *Cytotoxic T cells* – mostly CD8 T cells
   (b) *Natural killer (NK) cells* – these are large granular lymphocytes, and are present in the non-immune host
   (c) *Lymphokine-activated killer (LAK) cells*: probably a subset of NK cells, as a result of cytokine activation.

2. **Antibody-dependent cellular cytotoxicity or ADCC**: virus-infected cells can also be lysed by T cells with Fc receptors for IgG, which bind to target cells coated with viral IgG bound to virus on cell surfaces. These cells include:
   (a) *Killer (K) cells* – mainly responsible for this type of cell destruction: they are lymphocytes and are present in non-immune as well as immune hosts
   (b) *Polymorphonuclear leucocytes*
   (c) *Activated macrophages*.

Cytokines

Cytokines are small protein molecules released by many cells, including lymphocytes and macrophages: they function as signals or mediators to activate, modulate and control the immune responses (and other activities) of cells. There are numerous cytokines, e.g. interferons (see below), interleukins and tumour necrosis factor: many act sequentially and interact with other cytokines. In addition to their role in the immune response, some have physiological functions such as tissue repair, differentiation and signalling activity in the CNS.

Interferons (see p. 169) are cytokines which act to render cells refractory to virus infection. There are three main classes, reflecting the cell of origin:

1. **Alpha**: originate in leucocytes
2. **Beta**: originate in fibroblasts
3. **Gamma**: originate in T lymphocytes.

Interferons have anti-proliferative activity on cells and the immune system, as well as inhibiting virus replication.

Characteristics of interferons:

1. **Host-specific**: so that only human interferon is fully active in human cells
2. **Wide antiviral spectrum**: most viruses are inhibited
3. **Induced** by viruses and nucleic acids
4. **Action**: both virus transcription and protein synthesis are prevented.

Interferons were long thought to be potentially ideal chemotherapeutic agents against viruses, but this potential has not been realized in practice. Side-effects (similar to those of pyrogens) have proved troublesome and despite undoubted clinical response with some viruses, applications are fairly restricted. However, interferon therapy is proving useful in the treatment of some forms of chronic hepatitis due to viruses.

2. Virus replication

Viruses have no metabolic activity of their own: they replicate by taking over the biochemical machinery of the host cell and redirecting it to the manufacture of virus components. This take-over is achieved by virus mRNA.

VIRUS GROWTH CYCLE

Takes place in seven stages:

1. *Adsorption*
   (a) to specific receptors on the cell plasma membrane
   (b) best at 37°C but also occurs – although slowly – at 4°C
   (c) enhanced by Mg^{++} or Ca^{++}
2. *Entry*
   (a) complex: probably by invagination of cell membrane round the virus particle, to enclose it in a pinocytotic vacuole
   (b) in the case of syncytia-producing viruses, by fusion of virus envelope with cell membrane
3. *Uncoating*
   (a) releases – or renders accessible – the virus nucleic acid or genome
   (b) cell enzymes (from lysosomes) strip off the virus protein coat
4. *Transcription*
   (a) the production of virus mRNA or replicative intermediates from the viral genome
   (b) carried out either by host cell or virus-specified enzyme
   (c) subject to complex control mechanisms:
      • patterns of transcription often differ before (early) and after (late) virus nucleic acid replication
      • many virus genomes contain promoters and enhancers that stimulate transcription

13

- primary transcripts are often spliced to remove intron sequences between expressed exons
- transcription sometimes overlaps, with different starting and/or termination points within one gene, to produce different proteins from the same nucleic acid sequence

(d) virus mRNA generally, but not invariably:
- contains leader sequences
- is capped at the 5′ end
- is polyadenylated at the 3′ terminus

5. *Synthesis of virus components*

(a) virus protein synthesis: virus mRNA is translated on cell ribosomes into two types of virus protein:
- structural – the proteins which make up the virus particle
- non-structural – not found in the particle, mainly enzymes for virus genome replication

(b) virus nucleic acid synthesis:
- new virus genomes are synthesized
- templates are either the parental genome or, in the case of single-stranded nucleic acid genomes, newly formed complementary strands
- most often by a virus-coded polymerase or replicase: in the case of some DNA viruses a cell enzyme carries this out

6. *Assembly*

(a) new virus genomes and proteins are assembled to form new virus particles

(b) may take place in cell nucleus, cytoplasm or (with most enveloped viruses) at the plasma membrane, which invests the new particle to form the virus envelope

7. *Release*

either by sudden rupture or by gradual extrusion (budding) of enveloped viruses through the cell membranes.

VIRUS GENOMES

Nucleic acid

- May be DNA or RNA
- Single- or double-stranded
- Intact or segmented
- Linear or circular.

Large viruses

- Have high molecular weight nucleic acid
- Code for many proteins
- Code for many of the enzymes involved in replication.

Small viruses

- Have low molecular weight nucleic acid
- Therefore have limited coding capacity
- Must use some of the cell enzymes for replication.

Infectivity

In the case of many viruses, the purified nucleic acid is *infectious* when applied to cells – i.e. without the capsid, nucleic acid on its own can infect a cell, to initiate a complete infectious cycle of virus replication.

Virus genomes of which the virions contain a transcriptase are *non-infectious*: this is because the process of nucleic acid extraction removes the virion transcriptase and mRNA cannot then be produced.

Properties

The properties of the main virus groups and their genomes are shown in Table 2.1.

Baltimore classification

This classifies viruses into six groups on the basis of their nucleic acid and mRNA production (Fig. 2.1).

BIOCHEMISTRY OF VIRUS REPLICATION

An extremely complex subject: a few simplified examples will be outlined here to highlight the main differences between the growth cycles of some representative groups of viruses.

Double-stranded DNA viruses

Examples: vaccinia, herpes simplex, adenovirus, papillomavirus. The principal steps in their growth cycle are detailed below and shown diagrammatically in Figure 2.2.

Table 2.1   Some properties of viruses and their genomes

Virus family	Example	Genome[a]	Transcriptase contained in virus particles
Pox	Vaccinia	DS DNA	+
Herpes	Herpes simplex	DS DNA	0
Adeno	Adenovirus	DS DNA	0
Papova	Papilloma	DS DNA	0
Hepadna	Hepatitis B[e]	DS DNA[e]	+[b]
Parvo	B19	SS DNA	0
Picorna	Poliovirus	SS RNA	0
Calici	SRSVs	SS RNA	0
Toga	Rubella	SS RNA	0
Corona	Coronavirus	SS RNA	0
Orthomyxo	Influenza A	SS RNA[c]	+
Paramyxo	Measles	SS RNA	+
Arena	Lassa fever	SS RNA[c]	+
Bunya	Crimean-Congo haemorrhagic fever	SS RNA[c]	+
Flavi	Yellow fever	SS RNA	0
Filo	Marburg	SS RNA	0
Rhabdo	Rabies	SS RNA	+
Retro	HIV-1	SS RNA[d]	+[b]
Reovirus	Rotavirus[c]	DS RNA[c]	+

[a]DS = double-stranded; SS = single-stranded
[b]reverse transcriptase
[c]segmented genome (arena 2, bunya 3, orthomyxo 8, reovirus 11 unique subunits)
[d]two identical subunits in the virion
[e]virion contains DNA polymerase and reverse transcriptase.

Transcription

Two main types of mRNA are produced:

1. **Early mRNA** – before virus DNA synthesis: codes mainly for enzymes required for DNA synthesis
2. **Late mRNA** – after virus DNA synthesis: codes mainly for structural proteins.

Virus DNA synthesis

Enzymes: many are involved but:

- the main DNA replicative enzyme is DNA-dependent DNA polymerase

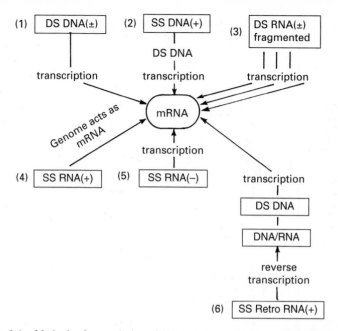

Fig. 2.1 Methods of transcription of the six different groups in the Baltimore classification of virus genomes. *Note*: (+) = positive-sense RNA, i.e. acts as a messenger; (−) = negative-sense RNA, i.e. transcribed to form complementary-sense strands, which then act as messengers.

- larger viruses (e.g. vaccinia, herpes simplex) code for their own enzyme
- smaller viruses (e.g. adenovirus, papillomavirus) use the host cell DNA polymerase.

Template: new progeny virus DNA is synthesized off the DNA genome of the input parental virus.

Site: nucleus (except poxviruses).

New progeny DNA: acts as templates for:

- transcription of late virus mRNA
- synthesis of more genomes for new virus particles.

Virus protein synthesis

This is a two-stage process:

1. **Production of early proteins** required for virus DNA synthesis (e.g. DNA-dependent DNA polymerase, thymidine kinase)

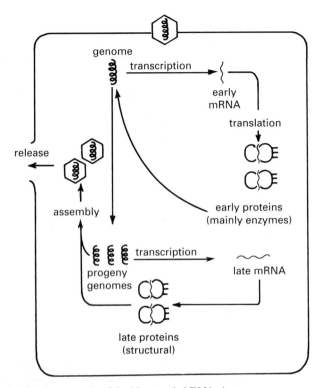

Fig. 2.2   Replicative cycle of double-stranded DNA virus.

2. *Production of late proteins*
- produced after virus DNA synthesis
- mostly the capsid proteins for new particles.

Site: virus proteins are synthesized on the ribosomes in the cell cytoplasm, and then transported to sites of assembly.

Assembly

Assembly of new DNA genomes and proteins into new infectious particles within the cell takes place in:

1. **Nucleus** (e.g. herpes simplex, adenovirus, papillomavirus)
   Note: herpes particles acquire an envelope by budding through the cell nuclear membrane, which has been modified by the incorporation within it of virus glycoproteins
2. **Cytoplasm**: vaccinia replicates entirely in the cytoplasm in 'factories' which are based on clusters of ribosomes.

Other DNA viruses

Hepatitis B virus has an unusual and complex replication cycle. The infectious particle contains an incompletely double-stranded DNA molecule and a DNA polymerase, which can fill in the gap to produce a complete double-stranded molecule. The polymerase also has reverse transcriptase activity. Replication of the genome is unique in that it involves production of an RNA template which then, by reverse transcription, synthesizes an RNA/DNA intermediate which is subsequently converted to double-stranded DNA. The genes for the surface and core proteins are overlapped by the gene for the DNA polymerase.

Parvoviruses have a tiny single-stranded DNA genome. Some are autonomous in replication (e.g. human parvovirus, B19); others are defective and require a helper virus for replication. B19 packages (in approximately equal proportions) both positive- and negative-strand DNA into virions, but separately within different particles.

RNA viruses

Because their genetic material is RNA, these viruses use biochemical mechanisms for their replication which are different from those of other forms of living organism. RNA virus genomes have different types of transcription:

1. **Single-strand positive-sense (plus-sense) RNA**: the virus genome is the virus mRNA
2. **Single-strand negative-sense (minus-sense) RNA**: virus mRNA is transcribed from the parental genome
3. **Double-stranded segmented RNA**: individual virus mRNAs are transcribed separately off the parental RNA segments using a transcriptase associated with each segment.

Retrovirus: a RNA virus whose genome alternates between RNA and DNA: virion single-stranded RNA is transcribed into double-stranded DNA, which is then integrated into the host chromosome as a 'provirus' from which virus RNA is later transcribed. But note, retrovirus genomes are inverted dimers of two complete genomes.

Below are selected examples of the replication cycle of some RNA viruses.

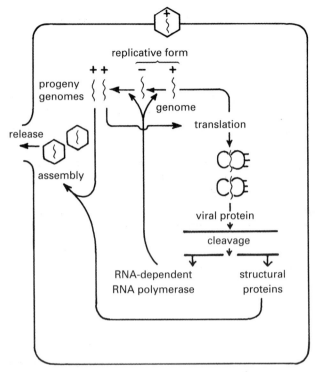

Fig. 2.3   Replicative cycle of single-strand positive-sense RNA virus.

Single-strand positive-sense RNA viruses

Example: poliovirus.

With these viruses, there is no transcription stage because the single-strand positive-sense genomic RNA itself acts as virus mRNA. The replication cycle is shown diagrammatically in Figure 2.3.

Translation

The virus genome is translated into one very large polypeptide, which is almost immediately cleaved into smaller proteins as follows:

1. Structural viral capsid proteins
2. The RNA-dependent RNA polymerase required for replication of virus RNA (no similar enzyme exists in cells)

3. A protease for cleaving the precursor polypeptide
4. A genome-linked terminal protein.

Virus RNA synthesis

New genome production takes place on a double-stranded 'replicative' form of RNA made by the synthesis of a negative-sense RNA strand complementary to the input positive-sense parental RNA.

New progeny positive-sense RNA strands are synthesized off the template of the negative RNA strand in the replicative form.

RNA-dependent RNA polymerase synthesizes both the replicative form and also new positive-sense RNA strand genomes.

Progeny positive-sense RNA functions as:

1. templates for the production of more replicative forms (and so for synthesis of more genome RNA)
2. genomes for new virus particles
3. virus mRNA.

Assembly

New progeny virus particles are assembled on clusters of ribosomes from the cleavage products of the primary translation product and from progeny virus RNA in the cytoplasm: poliovirus replicates entirely in the cytoplasm.

Release

By sudden rupture of the cell.

Single-strand negative-sense RNA viruses

Example: parainfluenza virus.

The replicative cycle is shown diagrammatically in Figure 2.4.

Transcription

Virus mRNA is synthesized off the parental (negative-sense strand) genome RNA using a transcriptase (RNA-dependent RNA polymerase) contained in the virus particle. Separate virus mRNAs are produced for each of the different virus proteins.

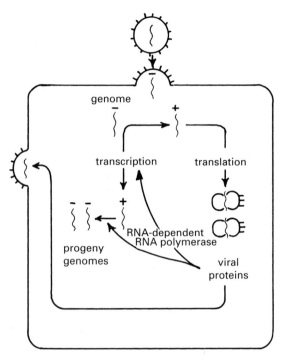

Fig. 2.4   Replicative cycle of single-strand negative-sense RNA virus.

Virus RNA synthesis

Virus progeny genomes are produced – also by the transcriptase – using positive-sense RNA strands complementary to the parental genome as templates.

Virus protein synthesis

Virus proteins include:

1. Transcriptase
2. Envelope proteins (two are glycosylated and have haemagglutinin/neuraminidase and fusion/haemolysis activities respectively)
3. Nucleocapsid proteins.

Assembly

New virus nucleocapsids are assembled at the cell membrane and become enveloped by budding through the plasma membrane.

Influenza virus

Influenza virus is unusual amongst single-stranded RNA viruses in that it has a segmented genome, each segment of which codes for a different virus protein.

New viral RNA is synthesized in the cell nucleus – a process that requires host cell transcription. Viral proteins are synthesized in the cytoplasm and migrate to the cell surface, where the envelope proteins become incorporated into the plasma membrane: new RNA genomes are also transported to the cell surface where they, with the newly synthesized viral proteins, are assembled into new virions. The virion envelope is acquired when the particles bud through the cell plasma membrane.

Double-stranded RNA viruses

Example: reoviruses.

All double-stranded RNA viruses have segmented genomes. Each segment codes for a different protein and each is associated with a molecule of transcriptase (RNA-dependent RNA polymerase).

The replicative cycle starts with transcription of mRNA from each double-stranded RNA segment – the mRNAs produced are then translated into the different virus proteins.

These mRNA molecules later become enclosed within nucleo-capsids, together with a transcriptase which directs the synthesis of a complementary RNA strand to produce the double-stranded segments which make up the genome.

Retroviruses

Example: HIV-1

Many – but not all – retroviruses are tumour viruses which can replicate in cells without killing them and can also transform normal cells into malignant or cancer cells. Their replication involves the production of virus DNA, which integrates into the cell chromosome.

The retrovirus genome is single-stranded dimeric RNA with three principal genes and with long terminal repeat regions which enable integration – in the DNA provirus form – into the host cell chromosome. The long terminal repeats contain promoter sequences. The three principal genes are:

1. *Gag*: core proteins

2. **Pol**: polymerase, i.e. reverse transcriptase (contained in the virion)
3. **Env**: envelope proteins.

Note: retroviruses contain several other genes with regulatory functions in viral replication.

The replicative cycle is shown diagrammatically in Figure 2.5.

First stage

1. **Transcription** (by the reverse transcriptase contained in the virion) to produce a DNA/RNA genome heteroduplex

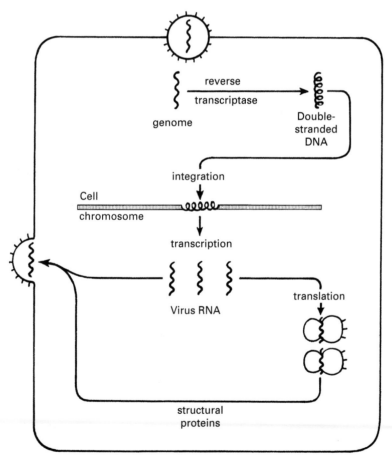

Fig. 2.5   Replicative cycle of retrovirus.

2. Conversion of the DNA/RNA heteroduplex into double-stranded DNA
3. Integration of the double-stranded virus DNA into the cellular chromosome, where it is known as *provirus*.

Second stage

1. Provirus DNA is transcribed (by cell enzyme)
2. The RNA transcripts produced have two functions:
   * mRNA for translation into virus proteins
   * new virus genomes.

Virus protein synthesis

Virus proteins are produced on cell ribosomes by translation of mRNA transcribed off the provirus DNA:

* Reverse transcriptase
* Core proteins
* Envelope proteins.

Assembly

Virus nucleocapsids are assembled from the progeny virus RNA genomes and proteins at the cell surface, and acquire their outer envelope by budding through the cell plasma membrane.

3. Laboratory diagnosis of virus infection

Virus diseases are diagnosed mainly by immunological techniques – that is, by demonstrating an antigen-antibody reaction to reveal evidence of virus infection.

Evidence of virus infection is shown by:

- Development of antibody to the virus at the time of or just after the symptoms of disease (serology)
- Presence of virus or virus products in the patient's blood or other tissues (virus isolation or direct demonstration of virus or viral components).

Automated technology (Fig. 3.1): has now largely – although not completely – replaced older and traditional methods of virus diagnosis. Automated technology:

1. is usually based on enzyme-linked immunosorbent assay (ELISA)
2. is sensitive, rapid, and economical of staff time
3. is carried out mainly using commercially-available kits (nowadays generally of good quality)
4. enables large numbers of patients to be diagnosed accurately and rapidly
5. detects IgM antibody, so that diagnosis can be made in the acute phase of illness.

SEROLOGY

Detection of virus-specific antibody, at the same time as (or shortly after) the symptoms of virus illness, is the most widely used method of diagnosis: ELISA is the commonest technique used.

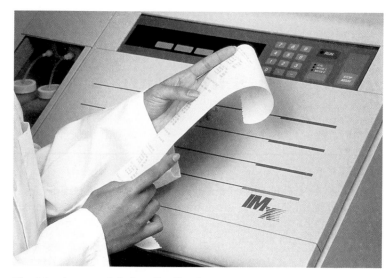

Fig. 3.1 Automated virology. Reading the computer-generated results printed out from an automated ELISA analyzer and reader. (Reproduced with the permission of Abbott Laboratories Ltd., Maidenhead, England.)

ELISA

The principles of ELISA are shown in Figure 3.2: note that demonstration of the diagnostic antigen-antibody reaction depends on:

1. Labelling antibody with enzyme, which reacts with an appropriate substrate to produce a measurable colour change.

2. A 'sandwich' technique (often used): patient's antibody reacting with a known virus is identified by addition of a second antibody, prepared in animals against the appropriate human immunoglobulin.

ELISAs can be varied by:

1. *Use of class-specific animal antibodies*: to detect IgM, IgG or IgA response to the virus.

2. *Competitive assay*: in which patient's serum competes with known (labelled) virus antibody for combining sites on the virus antigen: inhibition of the activity of the known antibody shows the presence of antibody in the patient's serum.

3. *Western blot*: in which virus proteins, separated on a cellulose membrane, are exposed to patient's serum: antibodies to individual proteins are detected to analyze the immune response

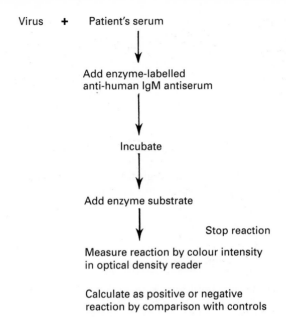

Virus + Patient's serum

Add enzyme-labelled
anti-human IgM antiserum

Incubate

Add enzyme substrate

Stop reaction

Measure reaction by colour intensity
in optical density reader

Calculate as positive or negative
reaction by comparison with controls

Fig. 3.2   ELISA test for virus IgM antibody.

to different virus structural proteins and therefore identify the stage and progress of the viral illness.

Other techniques

Other techniques used in serological diagnosis are described below.

Immunofluorescence

The label used is fluorescein dye: the immune reaction can be detected under UV light using a special microscope: liable to subjective interpretation and labour-intensive, but widely used.

Radioimmunoassay (RIA)

The label used is a radioisotope: sensitive and can be automated, but requires special conditions in the laboratory for handling radioactivity safely: therefore unsuitable for the average diagnostic laboratory.

Complement fixation test

When antigen reacts with antibody, complement (contained in guinea pig serum) is used up or 'fixed'. After addition of an indicator system such as red blood cells with anti-red-cell antibody, the red cells lyse if complement is present: that is, absence of haemolysis indicates a positive reaction (Fig. 3.3).

Haemagglutination-inhibition

Antiviral antibody blocks the agglutination of red cells by haemagglutinating viruses: strain-specific and mainly used in reference laboratories.

Radial haemolysis

The technique of *single radial haemolysis* is related to haemagglutination-inhibition. It detects antibody qualitatively by the appearance in agar gel of haemolysis round wells containing patients' sera. The gel contains red cells, virus and complement.

Neutralization

Antibody blocks viral infectivity in the case of cell cultures (and

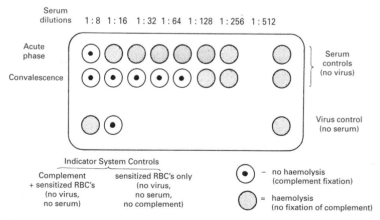

Fig. 3.3   Complement fixation test for viral antibody. Virus antigen is mixed overnight at 4°C with dilutions of the patient's serum and complement before the addition of sensitized sheep erythrocytes. Titre of complement-fixing antibody has risen from 8 in the acute phase to 128 in convalescence – a greater than 4-fold rise in titre, indicating recent infection.

laboratory animals): laborious and slow but still sometimes necessary.

Interpreting the significance of virus antibody

Virus antibodies (particularly IgG) are common in healthy populations and usually remain at a high level for many years after infection. A diagnosis of recent infection depends on the following criteria:

1. *Detection of IgM*: the earliest antibody to appear, and therefore only present if there has been recent infection. Now widely used as a method of rapid diagnosis: only one blood sample is required.

2. *Rising titre*: increase in the level of IgG antibody (at least four-fold) over the course of infection from the acute phase into convalescence (about 10 days). *Titre* is the highest dilution of an antiserum at which activity is demonstrated: usually expressed as the reciprocal of the antiserum dilution, e.g. 64 rather than 1/64.

3. *High stationary titre of IgG*: unreliable, but if the titre of antibody is considerably higher than that found in the general population, recent infection with the virus can be assumed.

Note: detection of virus IgG is often used to demonstrate pre-existing immunity or successful response to vaccination.

VIRUS: DIRECT TESTS

Antibodies tend to develop after the acute phase of infection, so detecting virus (or viral nucleic acid or proteins) is often a rapid way to diagnose virus infection in the laboratory.

Direct tests for virus include:

1. Antigen tests
2. Polymerase chain reaction (PCR)
3. Probes
4. Electron microscopy
5. Inclusion bodies.

Antigen tests

1. *ELISA*: basically the same method as that designed for antibody tests but adapted for antigen, for example by adsorbing

antibody to the wells of the test plate to 'capture' the virus: mono-clonal antibodies which have higher specificity are often used for this.

2. *Immunofluorescence*: fluorescein-labelled antibody detects virus antigen and enables the extent, localization within cells and distribution to be visualized.

Polymerase chain reaction (PCR) (Fig. 3.4)

A powerful molecular technique: exquisitely sensitive, and, in trained hands, highly specific: detects viral nucleic acid, DNA or RNA – the latter after a preliminary step of reverse transcription to produce complementary DNA off the RNA template. Now being widely used for diagnosis and for estimation of viral load.

Probes

Radiolabelled virus DNA sequences used to detect virus genome or mRNA in tissues and fluids by molecular hybridization.

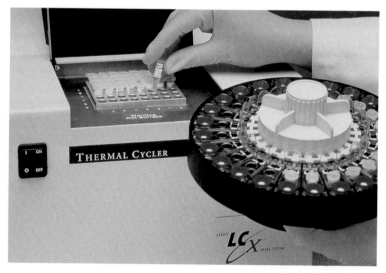

Fig. 3.4 Thermal cycler used for PCR: this allows the accurate temperature control needed for the synthesis of DNA by the thermostable enzyme Taq polymerase. DNA is denatured at high temperatures, alternating with cycles at lower temperatures for primer binding and the synthesis of specified regions of the DNA undergoing amplification. (Reproduced with the permission of Abbott Laboratories Ltd., Maidenhead, England.)

Electron microscopy

Laborious and insensitive (10^6 particles per ml are necessary for detection) but still required, for example, for the diagnosis of some faecal viruses and for detecting virus in vesicle fluid.

Inclusion bodies

Virus-induced masses seen in the nucleus or cytoplasm of infected cells in stained preparations: with a few exceptions, e.g. rabies, too nonspecific to be useful in diagnosis.

VIRUS ISOLATION

Virus isolation requires the use of living cells, since viruses cannot grow on inanimate media. Now used for diagnosis less than formerly. There are three main systems:

1. Tissue culture
2. Chick embryo
3. Laboratory animals } rarely used.

Tissue culture

Tissue culture is really cell culture in vitro, and consists of a single layer (monolayer) of actively metabolizing cells adherent to a glass or plastic surface in a test-tube or Petri plate, or on one side of a bottle.

The main types of tissue culture are:

1. ***Primary cultures***, e.g. monkey kidney: laborious to prepare and short-lived, but susceptible to a wide range of viruses.

2. ***Semi-continuous cell strains***, e.g. human embryo lung: easy to maintain and can be subcultured for about 20–30 passages before the cells die off. Susceptible to a wide range of viruses.

3. ***Continuous cell lines***, e.g. HeLa cells (derived from human cervical cancer): can be subcultured indefinitely and are therefore easy to maintain. Generally susceptible to fewer viruses than other types of cell culture.

Medium: cells are grown in balanced and buffered salt solutions with added amino acids, vitamins and serum. Antibiotics are included to prevent bacterial contamination.

Atmosphere: tissue cultures are grown in stoppered test tubes or screw-capped bottles or, if in Petri plates, in an incubator with the atmosphere enriched with 5–10% carbon dioxide.

Temperature: optimal temperature for cells is 37°C, but for some viruses 33°C is required.

Specimens: material from lesions or sites of infection can be conveniently collected on a wooden-shafted swab. The tip of the swab is broken off into a bottle of transport medium. Virus laboratories supply these on request.

Delivery: should be prompt as many viruses die off rapidly at room temperature. If delay is unavoidable, keep the specimen at 4°C (e.g. in a domestic refrigerator).

Inoculation: a small volume of virus in transport medium, vesicle or other fluid, or an extract in buffer solution of tissue or excretion, is added to the medium of a tube of tissue culture.

Virus growth

Virus growth is recognized by:

1. **CPE** (cytopathic effect): the virus kills the cells, which round up and fall off the glass (Fig. 3.5). Some viruses cause cell fusion, and their growth is recognized by the appearance of syncytia.

2. **Haemadsorption**: added erythrocytes adhere to the surface of cells infected with haemagglutinating virus (Fig. 3.6): some-

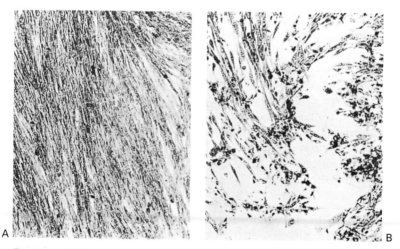

Fig. 3.5 CPE in a tissue culture of fibroblastic cells. (A) Uninoculated control; (B) Culture showing viral CPE.

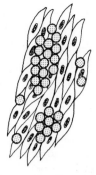

Fig. 3.6 Haemadsorption: clumps of erythrocytes are adhering to infected cells in the tissue culture.

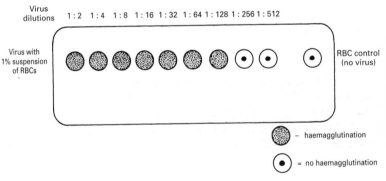

Fig. 3.7 Haemagglutination test for virus. Titre of virus haemagglutinin is 128.

times virus can be detected by haemagglutination in the medium (Fig. 3.7).

3. *Immunofluorescence*: infected cells are detected by fluorescence.

Identification: the virus isolated is identified serologically by neutralization of the CPE (or by inhibition of haemadsorption or haemagglutination) with standard antiviral serum or by immunofluorescence (with standard or monoclonal viral antibody). Electron microscopy is also occasionally used.

Chick embryo

Rarely used now for virus diagnosis. Useful for preparation of bulk virus, e.g. for antigen or vaccine production.

Laboratory animals

Some viruses can only be isolated by inoculation of laboratory animals, usually mice. After inoculation the animals are observed for signs of disease or death. The viruses are identified by testing for neutralization of their pathogenicity for the animals by standard sera.

4. Influenza

Influenza is the most important of the great epidemic diseases. From time to time, influenza becomes pandemic and sweeps throughout the world. The most severe pandemic recorded was in the winter of 1918–19, when more than 20 million people perished. World-wide pandemics of influenza are due to the emergence of antigenically new strains of influenza virus.

Clinical features

Transmission: inhalation of respiratory secretions from an infected person.

Incubation period: 1–4 days.

Symptoms: fever, malaise, headaches, generalized aches, a characteristic non-productive hacking cough: sometimes with sore throat and hoarseness, nasal discharge and sneezing.

Duration: symptoms usually last for about 4 days, but tiredness and weakness often persist for longer.

Primary site of virus multiplication: superficial epithelium of the lower respiratory tract. Influenza causes damage to the cilia and desquamation of the epithelium.

Complications

Two kinds of pneumonia may follow influenza:

1. *Primary influenzal pneumonia* is rare (but less rare in pandemics): a patient with typical influenza suddenly deteriorates, with the onset of severe respiratory distress and symptoms of hypoxia, dyspnoea and cyanosis; circulatory collapse follows and the patient almost always dies. Sometimes the onset is so sudden that typical signs of influenza have not developed. Post-mortem, there is congestion of the lungs with desquamation of ciliated

37

epithelium and hyperaemia of tracheal and bronchial mucosa; no significant bacteria are present.

2. **Secondary bacterial pneumonia** is more common, especially in the elderly or in patients with pre-existing cardiac or pulmonary disease: due to secondary invasion of the lungs by bacteria such as *Staphylococcus aureus, Haemophilus influenzae* or pneumococci. The signs and symptoms are those of severe bacterial pneumonia. Although there is a high case fatality rate, the disease is less lethal than primary influenzal pneumonia. Post-mortem, there is heavy invasion of the lungs by bacteria.

3. **Reye's syndrome**: (see also Chapter 6) a very rare complication seen in children after influenza (and other virus infections): neurological signs are prominent, with cerebral oedema and fatty degeneration of the viscera, especially the liver, which results in raised transaminase levels in the blood. The mortality is 20–35%. Aspirin predisposes to the syndrome and children should not be treated with this drug unless there are special indications.

Types of virus

There are three influenza viruses: A, B and C, differentiated antigenically by their internal nucleoprotein (see below):

- *A*: the principal cause of epidemic influenza
- *B*: usually a milder disease but also causes winter outbreaks (especially in children)
- *C*: of doubtful pathogenicity for humans.

Influenza A viruses are also found in animals – notably birds, pigs and horses.

Epidemiology

Seasonal distribution: most prevalent during the winter (but the pandemic of 'Asian' influenza started in Britain in the summer of 1957): influenza is present every winter in temperate climates. This seasonal prevalence is much less marked in tropical countries.

Spread: more rapid than with any other infectious disease: influenza virus possesses an inherent capacity for rapid spread.

Epidemics: pandemics of influenza A break out every few years and the epidemic strain spreads world-wide. The epidemic in 1918–19 was due to a virus related to swine influenza A virus;

unlike influenza outbreaks in recent years, this caused a high mortality amongst young adults. Influenza nowadays is most severe in the elderly or in patients with chronic respiratory or cardiac disease.

Epidemic spread: is associated with antigenic change in the haemagglutinin on the virus surface – the main antigen involved in virus neutralization. This may be due to radical change in the haemagglutinin – *antigenic shift* – or, more commonly, progressive (if less dramatic) *antigenic drift* (see below).

Virology

1. Orthomyxoviruses ('myxo' = affinity for mucin).

2. RNA viruses: the single-strand negative-sense RNA is in eight separate segments, each of which is a gene and codes for a different protein, e.g. the haemagglutinin, the neuraminidase, etc.

3. Roughly spherical particles, medium size, 80–100 nm, with an envelope which contains radially-projecting spikes of virus hae-magglutinin and neuraminidase (Fig. 4.1). Inside the envelope is a helically-coiled nucleocapsid, consisting of RNA surrounded by protein capsomeres.

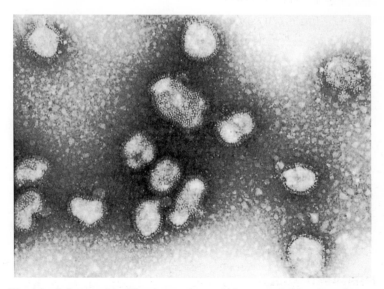

Fig. 4.1   Influenza virus. The virus nucleocapsid is surrounded by an envelope containing spikes of haemagglutinin and neuraminidase. × 90 000. (Photograph by Dr E A C Follett.)

4. Haemagglutinate erythrocytes of various animal species.

5. Grow in monkey kidney tissue culture with haemadsorption; in amniotic cavity of the chick embryo and – after passage or subculture – in the allantoic cavity also.

Antigenic structure

Influenza viruses have three main antigens:

1. *'S' or soluble antigen*: the protein in the ribonucleoprotein core of the virus particle. All influenza A viruses share a common 'S' antigen which is different from that present in all influenza B viruses; demonstrated by complement fixation test.

2. *Haemagglutinin*: contained in the radially-projecting spikes in the virus envelope; strain-specific: the main neutralizing antigen responsible for immunity to the virus.

3. *Neuraminidase*: also antigenic and contained in the virus envelope; plays a minor role in immunity to reinfection.

Haemagglutination by influenza viruses

Influenza viruses have two proteins embedded in the surface envelope:

1. *Haemagglutinin*: the spikes on the surface that combine with specific receptors on the erythrocyte surface: these receptors are composed of sialic acid, a mucopolysaccharide – neuraminic acid.

2. *Neuraminidase*: a sialidase: an enzyme which destroys the neuraminic acid receptors on erythrocytes. At 37°C, the neuraminidase becomes active and causes elution of the virus from the erythrocytes; as a result the haemagglutination is reversed and the erythrocytes disperse again.

Haemagglutination inhibition: specific antibody prevents virus haemagglutination; haemagglutination inhibition is strain-specific, so that the antigenic variation in a new strain of virus can be measured by the decrease in the haemagglutination-inhibiting activity of antibody to the older strain.

Influenza A

Influenza A viruses are uniquely able to undergo frequent antigenic change. Epidemics are due to the emergence of a new virus strain containing a haemagglutinin (and sometimes a neuraminidase also) different from those of previously circulating viruses, so that the population has diminished immunity (i.e. lacks antibody) to the new haemagglutinin. Antigenic change may be:

- **major**: antigenic *shift*
- **minor**: antigenic *drift*.

Antigenic shift

This involves the replacement (by genetic reassortment) of the RNA segment which codes for the haemagglutinin by one from a different, possibly animal, virus strain. This can take place when two different influenza viruses infect and replicate in the same cell. As a result, a new virus emerges which has a novel haemagglutinin (to which human populations have no pre-existing antibody) and which can therefore spread pandemically. The same mechanism of genetic reassortment can also result in the acquisition of a novel neuraminidase.

Table 4.1 lists the main (shifted) influenza A viruses of the last 80 years.

Table 4.1 Main influenza A viruses

Year of emergence	Haemagglutinin	Neuraminidase
1918	H1	N1
1957	H2	N2
1968	H3	N2

Antigenic drift

Antigenic drift is due to spontaneous mutations in the haemagglutinin gene, causing minor substitutions in the amino acid sequence of the haemagglutinin protein (although the haemagglutinin remains basically the same protein). The drifted strain of virus then becomes selected in the population by virtue of its ability to infect partially immune hosts. Antigenic drift increases progressively from season to season.

Epidemics

Several pandemics of influenza have been recorded this century:

- 1918–19: due to an H1N1 swine influenza strain. This virus was never isolated, but its antigenic structure has been deduced from analyses of stored sera collected at the time and from genetic analysis of RNA recovered by PCR from stored lung tissue of fatal cases in the pandemic.
- 1933: the first influenza virus (a drifted H1N1 strain) was isolated.
- 1957: H2N2: the 'Asian flu' epidemic.
- 1968: H3N2: the 'Hong Kong flu' epidemic.
- 1977: H1N1 reappeared: 'Red flu' a mild form of influenza that infected young people, because older people had antibody from exposure to the virus before 1957.
- 1989: H3N2 caused a widespread epidemic, with many deaths, in the UK in late 1989 after many years of low influenza activity.

Since 1977 both H3N2 and H1N1 strains (interspersed with B strains) have circulated together in countries throughout the world (but there has been considerable antigenic drift, particularly in the case of H3N2).

Influenza B

Influenza B also shows antigenic variation, but the changes are less dramatic than in the case of influenza A. The following strains have been identified:

- 1973: a new strain, B/Hong Kong, appeared
- 1979: B/Singapore appeared
- 1988: B/Yamagata appeared
- At present: the current B strain is drifted from B/Yamagata.

Diagnosis

Direct demonstration:
  Specimen: nasopharyngeal aspirate.
  Detect virus antigen by indirect immunofluorescence: a very rapid method of diagnosis.
  Serology: (widely used):
  Complement fixation test: with the 'S' or soluble nucleoprotein antigen.
  Isolation:
  Specimen: nasopharyngeal aspirates are best – otherwise throat or nasal swabs.
  Inoculate: monkey kidney tissue cultures.

Observe: for haemagglutination or haemadsorption with human group O erythrocytes.

Type virus: by complement fixation: strain identification by haemagglutination-inhibition in a reference laboratory.

Vaccination

Vaccination is currently recommended for those suffering from cardiac or respiratory problems especially if elderly. This is to protect those at high risk of death or serious complications. Vaccination is not aimed at preventing transmission, and cannot do so.

In a pandemic, the speed with which new strains of influenza virus spread makes it difficult, if not impossible, to prepare sufficient quantities of vaccine in time to protect more than a few key workers.

Virus vaccine

Contains: inactivated virus grown in chick embryos: either purified subunits (i.e. surface antigen) or disrupted virus purified and ether-treated to solubilize envelope proteins.

Current vaccine: contains three strains:

- Influenza A, H1N1 and H3N2
- Influenza B.

Administration: intramuscularly, annually.

Protection: relatively short-lived (around a few months): effective but not solid immunity (around 60% protection) conferred.

Contraindicated: in people allergic to egg protein; pregnant women.

Complications: *Guillain-Barré syndrome*: a polyneuritis with ascending paralysis, usually starting in the legs, is a rare complication of influenza vaccination: clears up spontaneously, although positive pressure respiration may be required during the acute phase due to paralysis of the respiratory muscles.

Live attenuated virus vaccines

Administration: intranasally: not yet generally accepted.

Prophylaxis and treatment: Amantadine (see Chap. 18) can protect against influenza (not influenza B) and is effective in treatment if given early in infection.

5. Other respiratory tract infections

Respiratory infections are the commonest illnesses seen in general practice. Most are due to viruses that infect both upper and lower respiratory tracts – often simultaneously. Predominantly upper respiratory syndromes usually show some involvement of the lower respiratory tract, and vice versa. This chapter describes the viruses (with the exception of influenza virus) which cause respiratory disease.

Transmission: rapid, by inhalation of respiratory secretions and by surface contamination (including hands) with nasal secretions.

The principal viruses which affect the respiratory tract are shown in Table 5.1.

Table 5.1 Viruses which affect the respiratory tract

Virus	No. of serotypes	Disease
Parainfluenza viruses	4	Croup, colds, lower respiratory infections in children
Respiratory syncytial virus	1	Bronchiolitis and pneumonia in infants, colds
Rhinoviruses	100+	Colds
Adenoviruses	47	Pharyngitis and conjunctivitis
Coronaviruses	3	Colds

PARAINFLUENZA VIRUSES

Clinical features

A wide spectrum of respiratory syndromes – from severe, life-threatening lower respiratory tract disease to mild, self-limiting upper respiratory infection:

1. *Croup or acute laryngotracheobronchitis*: particularly associated with parainfluenza type 1: seen mainly in infants and young children; preceded by symptoms of a common cold, which worsen with increasing hoarseness, cough and the development of severe inspiratory stridor – which can lead to respiratory distress and cyanosis requiring tracheostomy.

2. *Common cold* with coryza, sore throat, hoarseness, cough and, sometimes, fever are features of parainfluenza infections, especially in older children and adults.

3. *Bronchiolitis and pneumonia* in young children are also sometimes caused by parainfluenza viruses – particularly type 3.

Immunocompromised: parainfluenza type 3 has a predilection for these patients: nosocomial outbreaks have been reported in bone marrow transplant units, where there is a high death rate – often due to giant cell pneumonia.

Age: affects both children and adults, but most common in children under 5 years old; the more severe infections are seen in pre-school children.

Serotypes

Four: types 1, 2, 3 and 4 – but type 4 is of lower pathogenicity.

Serotypes and disease: although there is considerable overlap, type 3 virus is particularly associated with bronchiolitis and bronchopneumonia and types 1 and 2 with croup. Type 3 infects younger children more than types 1 and 2.

Epidemiology

Type 3 tends to be endemic in the community, with a peak incidence in the spring. Types 1 and 2 used to be seen every second year, sometimes together, but this pattern has been less clear in recent years.

Immunity is not long-lasting and reinfections are common.

Virology

1. Paramyxoviruses
2. RNA viruses: single-strand negative-sense RNA
3. Large enveloped particles, 100–200 nm, with helical symmetry and possessing both haemagglutinin and neuraminidase
4. Haemagglutinate human group O erythrocytes
5. Grow in monkey kidney tissue cultures with haemadsorption.

Diagnosis

Direct demonstration of virus in nasopharyngeal aspirates by immunofluorescence.

Isolation:

Specimens: mouth washings, throat swabs.

Inoculate: monkey kidney tissue cultures.

Observe: for haemadsorption (CPE is variable and slow) or immunofluorescence.

Type virus: by neutralization test of haemadsorption by standard antisera.

Serology: of little value.

RESPIRATORY SYNCYTIAL VIRUS

Respiratory syncytial virus causes common colds, but its importance lies in its tendency to invade the lower respiratory tract in infants under 1 year old, causing bronchiolitis or pneumonia.

Clinical features

Incubation period: average 5 days, but range is 2–8 days.

Colds: the most common manifestation of infection: usually seen in children, especially in those under 5 years old, but sometimes affects the elderly (also with lower respiratory involvement).

Bronchiolitis: is seen in infants, especially in the first 6 months of life: starts with nasal obstruction and discharge (i.e. the symptoms of a common cold), but this is followed by fever, cough, rapid breathing, expiratory wheezes and signs of respiratory distress, such as cyanosis and inspiratory indrawing of the intercostal spaces.

Pneumonia: also mainly seen in small infants: the clinical picture is similar to that of bronchiolitis with fever, cyanosis, prostration and rapid breathing, but without expiratory wheezing.

Bronchiolitis and pneumonia are life-threatening, with a mortality of 2–5%.

Virus shedding: infected children are infectious, i.e. they shed virus in respiratory secretions, for 3–8 days.

Immunopathology

Inactivated vaccine against this virus enhanced the incidence of bronchiolitis and pneumonia in vaccinees compared to controls: this suggested that there may be an immunological component of the pathology of the disease in infants – in whom maternal antibodies would still be present, possibly causing formation of immune complexes. Alternatively, the susceptibility of very young infants may be mechanical, due to the narrowness of the bronchiolar lumen: when this is inflamed, there may be serious obstruction not seen in older infants with wider bronchioles.

Epidemiology

Every year there are outbreaks of respiratory syncytial virus, most often during the winter months from December to March.

Virology

1. Pneumovirus: a paramyxovirus: one serological type, but with some strain variation
2. RNA virus: single-strand negative-sense RNA
3. Pleomorphic enveloped particles, medium size, 90–130 nm; helical symmetry (Fig. 5.1)
4. Grows in cells with syncytial CPE
5. Does not haemagglutinate.

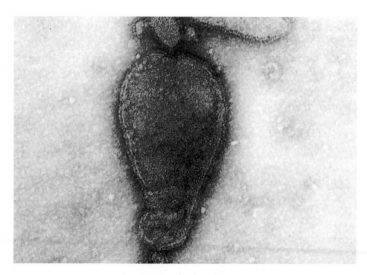

Fig. 5.1   Respiratory syncytial virus. Pleomorphic virus with helical nucleocapsid surrounded by an envelope. × 90 000. (Photograph by Dr E A C Follett.)

Diagnosis

Direct demonstration of virus in nasopharyngeal aspirates by immunofluorescence: now the most widely used method.

Isolation:

Specimens: mouth washings, nasal secretions (not frozen during delivery, because the virus is inactivated by freezing).

Inoculate: HEp-2 cells; HeLa cells.

Observe: for characteristic syncytial CPE of giant cells.

Type virus: by immunofluorescence or by complement fixation test.

Serology: complement fixation test: now little used.

Treatment

Ribavirin: (see Chap. 18) administered by inhalation in a special hood is effective in the treatment of severe infection. High-titred respiratory syncytial virus immunoglobulin also shows promise in early trials.

RHINOVIRUSES

Rhinoviruses cause roughly a third of common colds.

Clinical features

Incubation period: 2–4 days.

Signs and symptoms: nasal discharge with nasal obstruction, sneezing, sore throat and cough; about half the patients are mildly febrile; hoarseness and headache are common, especially in adults.

Duration: symptoms subside in about a week on average, but are prolonged for up to 2 weeks in some cases.

Complications: include sinusitis and otitis media.

Transmission: most common in the home or in school: rhinoviruses spread by contact (i.e. from hand to nose) as well as by inhalation of respiratory secretions: rhinoviruses can survive for some hours on skin or other surfaces.

Age: most frequent in pre-school children: thereafter the attack rate falls, but infections are common even amongst adults.

Incidence: variable, but on average the attack rate is about one rhinovirus infection per person per year.

Seasonal prevalence: infections are found all year round, but are most common in autumn and spring.

Immunity

Neutralizing antibody is formed after rhinovirus infection, in both blood and respiratory secretions: respiratory IgA shows the main protective effect against reinfection with the particular serotype responsible. The large number of serotypes, however, gives opportunity for frequent (new) infections.

Epidemiology

This is complex, as would be expected from the numerous virus serotypes. In any community at a given time, several serotypes can be found circulating; over a period of time, however, there is a gradual change in the serotypes present, probably due to increasing immunity within the population to earlier serotypes.

Virology

1. Picornaviruses (pico = small + RNA); more than 100 serotypes
2. RNA viruses, single-strand positive-sense RNA
3. Small, icosahedral particles, 22–30 nm
4. Inactivated at acid pH (unlike the enteroviruses – the other members of the picornavirus group)
5. Grow in human embryo cells, but at 33°C, instead of the usual 37°C (some also grow in monkey kidney cells).

Diagnosis

Isolation:

   Specimens: nasal secretions, mouth washings.
   Inoculate: human embryo lung and monkey kidney cell cultures.
   Observe: for CPE.
   Type virus: by neutralization with standard antisera.
   Note: culture of specimens for rhinoviruses is not routinely carried out in virus laboratories and it is rare for isolates to be typed. This is a pity, as it has hampered epidemiological research.

ADENOVIRUSES

Respiratory infection: clinical features

Clinically, the main symptoms of adenovirus respiratory infection are pharyngitis and conjunctivitis. The main syndromes are classified as shown in Table 5.2.

Table 5.2   Respiratory syndromes associated with adenoviruses

Syndrome	Adenovirus types
1. *Epidemic infection* Pharyngoconjunctival fever, acute respiratory disease	3, 4, 7, 14, 21
2. *Endemic infection* Pharyngitis, follicular conjunctivitis	1, 2, 5, 6
3. *Epidemic keratoconjunctivitis or 'shipyard eye'*	8, 19, 37

Epidemic infection: seen in army recruit camps, where attack rates of 70% have been reported, and in children's institutions, due to crowding together of susceptible young hosts.

Endemic infection: adenovirus infections are endemic, but at low level, in the general population: they usually constitute at most around 3% of the respiratory infections in the community at large. Types 1, 2, 5 and 6 are associated with endemic infection, but cases of infection due to types 3 and 7 are common in the community and tend to be found in clusters.

Epidemic keratoconjunctivitis: a form of eye infection which is spread by contaminated instruments at eye clinics and surgeries; epidemics are seen in eye patients, and also in shipyard and metal workers who are prone to minor eye injuries which require treatment at eye clinics: the disease is mainly associated with adenovirus type 8, although other types have been reported.

Faecal adenoviruses: adenoviruses are often found in the intestine during respiratory infection. However, certain types (40 and 41) cause viral gastroenteritis: these viruses are 'fastidious' and do not grow in routine cell cultures (see Ch. 7).

Other syndromes

Alimentary tract: faecal adenoviruses probably play a role in mesenteric adenitis and intussusception in children.

Bone marrow transplantation: adenovirus infection, sometimes disseminated, has been reported in recipients of transplants: AIDS patients are also vulnerable to severe adenovirus infection.

Acute haemorrhagic cystitis: has also been described associated, but not exclusively, with adenovirus type 11.

Persistent infection: adenoviruses have a tendency to persist for long periods in tissues such as the tonsils, adenoids and, less

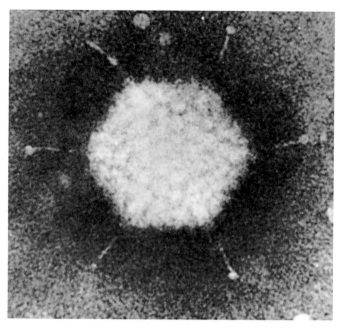

Fig. 5.2   Adenovirus. Icosahedron-shaped particle with cubic symmetry and fibres which project from the vertices. × 200 000. (Reproduced, with permission, from Valentine R C, Pereira H G 1965 Journal of Molecular Biology 13: 13.)

often, kidneys: this may not be true latency, but rather a low grade chronic infection.

Oncogenic properties: several adenoviruses cause cancer on injection into hamsters: the most highly oncogenic are types 12, 18 and 31. However, adenoviruses do not cause tumours in humans.

Virology

1. The different serological types react independently in neutralization tests, but share a common group complement-fixing antigen
2. Double-stranded DNA viruses
3. Medium size: 60–70 nm; icosahedron-shaped particles with cubic symmetry and with fibres topped with knobs projecting from the vertices (Fig. 5.2)
4. Most haemagglutinate

5. Grow slowly in tissue cultures (human embryonic cells or HeLa cells are best) with CPE of clusters of rounded, 'ballooned' cells.

Diagnosis

Isolation:

Specimens: mouth washings, throat swabs, faeces.

Inoculate: human embryonic cell cultures or HeLa cells.

Observe: for characteristic CPE of large rounded cells like 'bunches of grapes'.

Type virus: by neutralization test.

Serology: complement fixation test detects antibody to adenovirus group antigen, but not the serotype of the adenovirus responsible.

Direct demonstration: electron microscopy or specialized cell culture is used for detection of fastidious adenoviruses in faeces.

OTHER VIRUSES CAUSING COMMON COLDS

Coronaviruses

Medium-sized (80–100 nm) single-stranded RNA, positive-sense viruses; characteristic enveloped particles surrounded by a fringe of club-shaped projections.

Haemagglutinate: can only be isolated in organ cultures of human embryo trachea, although some strains, notably 229E, have been adapted to growth in the L 132 line of human embryo lung cells with CPE. At least three antigenic types.

Coronaviruses cause around 10% of colds in the community. Difficult to isolate in the laboratory: diagnose by serology.

Toroviruses: similar to coronaviruses and found in the stools of children (and adults) with diarrhoea, but their role in this is uncertain.

Enteroviruses

Enteroviruses also cause respiratory infections – such infections associated with a variety of echoviruses and coxsackieviruses have been reported.

6. Neurological diseases due to viruses

Viruses are important causes of neurological disease – most often as a complication of infection elsewhere in the body.

Spread: most viruses invade the CNS via the blood stream, but some (e.g. rabies) reach the CNS by the neural route, by spread along peripheral nerves.

Virus neurological diseases can be classified as:

1. Acute virus infections of the CNS
2. Chronic virus neurological disease
3. Neurological syndromes precipitated by virus infection.

ACUTE VIRUS INFECTIONS OF THE CNS

There are two main clinical syndromes:

1. *Aseptic meningitis*: generally a mild disease with complete recovery, symptoms are fever, headache and stiffness of neck and back: can sometimes progress to asymmetric, flaccid, lower motor neurone paralysis (*poliomyelitis*), which can result in permanent disability.

2. *Encephalitis*: symptoms are drowsiness, mental confusion, convulsions, and focal neurological signs, leading to stupor and sometimes coma.

Table 6.1 summarizes the features of acute viral neurological disease.

CHRONIC VIRUS NEUROLOGICAL DISEASES

Viruses and prions cause several chronic neurological diseases, which are listed in Table 6.2 and are described in more detail in later chapters.

Table 6.1 Acute virus neurological diseases

Disease	Asetic meningitis	Encephalitis	
		Primary	Post-infectious
Lesions	Meningeal inflammation occasionally progresses to destruction of anterior horn cells	Varied: perivascular cuffing; changes may be necrotizing (herpes simplex) or minimal (rabies): inclusions often present	Multifocal perivenous demyelination
Pathogenesis	Direct invasion of brain by virus	Direct invasion of brain by virus	Probably immunological: follows 2–14 days after acute disease or vaccination
CSF	Virus often present Lymphocytes ++	No virus Lymphocytes +	No virus Lymphocytes +
Viruses	Enteroviruses, mumps	Herpes simplex, mumps, arthropod-borne viruses, rabies	Measles, rubella, varicella, vaccinia, rabies immunization

Table 6.2 Chronic virus neurological diseases

Disease	Subacute sclerosing panencephalitis	Progressive multifocal leucoencephalopathy	Creutzfeldt-Jakob disease, kuru	Tropical spastic paraparesis	HIV dementia/ encephalopathy
Site	Brain	Brain	Brain and spinal cord	Thoracic spinal cord	Brain
Lesions	Neuronal degeneration, intra-nuclear inclusions	Multiple foci of demyelination	Spongiform degeneration	Degeneration, perivascular cuffing	Cerebral atrophy and degenerative change
Infectious agents	Measles, congenital rubella	JC virus	Prions	HTLV-I	HIV-1 and 2

Chronic neurological diseases due to viruses and prions have the following features in common:

- Onset is gradual
- Symptoms are varied but are always severe and progressive
- The diseases (except for HTLV-I spastic paraparesis) are virtually always fatal.

NEUROLOGICAL SYNDROMES PRECIPITATED BY VIRUS INFECTION

Two important neurological diseases can be associated with virus infections, although the mechanism of induction is unclear and there are almost certainly non-infective factors involved.

Reye's syndrome

A disease characterized by fatty degeneration of CNS and liver: seen only in children: aspirin increases the risk of developing the disease.
Clinical features:

1. Usually follows 4–6 weeks after a virus infection
2. Nausea and vomiting with CNS symptoms progressing from lethargy, mental change, convulsions, to coma; hepatomegaly
3. Mortality is high – case fatality rate around 10–40%.

Cause: associated with various virus infections – influenza B, varicella, less often influenza A, rarely a variety of other viruses.

Guillain-Barré syndrome

An acute demyelinating polyneuropathy involving the peripheral nerves; probably immunologically-mediated; seen at all ages.
Clinical features:

1. Approximately two-thirds of patients have had a viral infection some 4–6 weeks before onset
2. Flaccid, symmetric paralysis of legs, sometimes ascending to involve muscles of respiration
3. Spontaneous recovery is usual but some patients may require assisted ventilation before the symptoms subside.

Cause: various viruses have been incriminated, including cytomegalovirus and EB (Epstein-Barr) virus – and influenza vaccination, although the virus in this vaccine is inactivated; can also follow surgery, and sometimes associated with lymphoma.

7. Enterovirus infections

Enteroviruses are a large group within the picorna family of viruses, which primarily infect the gut: surprisingly, they rarely cause intestinal symptoms: enterovirus diseases are the result of spread of the viruses to other sites of the body – particularly the CNS.

Table 7.1 lists the various viruses included in the enterovirus family.

Enteroviruses have the following properties:

1. Enter the body via ingestion by mouth
2. Primary site of multiplication is the lymphoid tissue of the alimentary tract – including the pharynx
3. Spread from the gut is in two directions:
   a. Outwards into the blood (viraemia) and so to other tissues and organs
   b. Inwards into the lumen of the gut and so to excretion into the faeces.

Table 7.1 Enteroviruses

	Polio-viruses	Coxsackieviruses* A	Coxsackieviruses* B	Echoviruses[†]	Enteroviruses (unclassified)
Types[+]	1–3	1–24	1–6	1–33	68–71

[+] The types are not entirely sequential e.g. the original coxsackie A23 and echovirus 28 have been classified as other viruses.

* Coxsackie is the village in New York where these viruses were first isolated.

[†] Enteric, Cytopathic, Human, Orphan (Orphan because originally – but wrongly – thought not to be associated with human disease).

Table 7.2   Enterovirus disease

Syndrome	Main viruses responsible
1. Neurological	
(i) Paralysis	(i) Polioviruses
(ii) Aseptic meningitis	(ii) Most enteroviruses
2. Febrile illness	Most enteroviruses
3. Herpanginas; hand, foot and mouth disease	Coxsackie A viruses
4. Myocarditis, pericarditis	Coxsackie B viruses
5. Bornholm disease	Coxsackie B viruses
6. Acute haemorrhagic conjunctivitis	Enterovirus 70, Coxsackievirus A24

Clinical features

The main enterovirus diseases are shown in Table 7.2.

General features of enterovirus infections

Most infections are confined to the alimentary tract and are symptomless: enteroviruses do not cause diarrhoea.

A small proportion of infections give rise to febrile illness due to viraemia.

Still fewer cases progress to aseptic meningitis and – more rarely still – to paralysis: spread of virus to the CNS or other organs and tissues is a relatively rare complication of enterovirus infection.

Neurological syndromes

Neurological disease is the most important manifestation of enteroviral infection; caused by many different types of enterovirus – although some enteroviruses are more prone to cause neurological symptoms than others.

The illness is usually biphasic: the initial symptoms are of febrile illness due to viraemia; there is an intervening period of well-being for a day or two, followed by the onset of neurological symptoms due to spread of the virus through the blood–brain barrier to invade the CNS.

There are two main neurological syndromes due to enteroviruses:

1. ***Aseptic meningitis***: is the more common; CNS damage is minor, with fever, headache and nuchal rigidity (stiffness of the neck muscles due to meningeal irritation). Lymphocytes and protein

in the cerebrospinal fluid (CSF) are increased. Most patients recover completely.

2. **Paralysis** (or *poliomyelitis*, because most often due to the polioviruses): an acute illness with pain and flaccid paralysis, generally affecting the lower legs. Sometimes bulbar paralysis, when the muscles of breathing and swallowing are involved. Paralysis is an extension of aseptic meningitis and is accompanied by the signs and symptoms of that syndrome.

Pathology: paralysis is due to viral damage to the cells of the anterior horn of the spinal cord, with lower motor neurone lesions resulting in flaccid paralysis. If damage to the nerve cells is severe, the paralysis becomes irreversible (Fig. 7.1).

Polioviruses: are the most paralytogenic enteroviruses – especially poliovirus type 1. Poliomyelitis was formerly common as infantile paralysis (and still is in some of the developing countries of the world), although sometimes involving adults in areas where infection was uncommon in childhood due to high standards of hygiene: however the disease has now been eliminated in many countries by vaccination.

Non-neurological syndromes

Febrile illness: a common manifestation of any enterovirus infection, and due to viraemia.

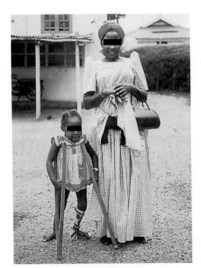

Fig. 7.1   Poliomyelitis. Child with residual paralysis and wasting in affected leg. (Photograph by Dr Eric Walker.)

Rash: many enteroviruses cause rash, but this is particularly common with coxsackieviruses A9 and A16 (see below) and echovirus 9.

Herpangina: typically a painful eruption of vesicles in the mouth and throat, but seen as part of the syndrome of hand, foot and mouth disease, in which there are vesicles also on the hands and feet; due to group A coxsackieviruses (especially A16); enterovirus 71 also causes hand, foot and mouth disease.

Bornholm disease: also known as *pleurodynia* or *epidemic myalgia*: a painful inflammation of the intercostal muscles. The disease is named after the Danish island where there was an extensive outbreak in 1930; due to group B coxsackieviruses.

Myocarditis and pericarditis: usually seen together and due to group B coxsackieviruses. Myocarditis is characterized by rapid pulse, enlargement of the heart and ECG abnormalities, and pericarditis by pericardial friction or effusion: seen mainly in adult males, and may be mistaken for myocardial infarction; however, most patients recover completely.

Acute haemorrhagic conjunctivitis: due to enterovirus 70 and a variant of coxsackievirus A24; appeared in large-scale outbreaks in 1969–71 in South East Asia and Africa, and has since been seen world-wide. The incubation period is 24 h and the disease lasts about 10 days: patients recover completely: the disease spreads rapidly, probably via eye discharges. Virus is usually found in the faeces only in the prodromal phase and not during the acute illness.

Epidemiology

Enterovirus infections are common, especially in children and in conditions of poor hygiene. In children in tropical or developing countries, multiple infection of the gut with several different viruses simultaneously is common.

Spread: mainly by the faecal–oral route from virus excretors to contacts; virus in pharyngeal secretions may also be a source of infection. High standard of living, in countries such as the USA, diminishes the chance of infection and therefore of immunity being acquired in childhood.

Gut immunity: after infection, the gut becomes resistant to reinfection with the same virus due to production in the gut of virus-specific neutralizing IgA antibody.

Seasonal distribution: infection is common in the summer months.

Epidemics of aseptic meningitis are seen, with one or sometimes two viruses predominating. Nowadays the epidemiology is more of sporadic infections, which increase in incidence during the summer months, and with several different viruses responsible. Echovirus 9 is often seen in outbreaks and, before the widespread use of polio vaccine, polioviruses were a major cause of epidemic aseptic meningitis. Echoviruses 4, 6, 11, 14, 16 and 30 and coxsackieviruses A9 and B5 also cause epidemic aseptic meningitis.

Epidemic poliomyelitis: before the advent of polio vaccines, countries with a high standard of living had a relatively high proportion of non-immune adults and suffered from repeated and widespread epidemics of paralytic disease, involving adults as well as children. Adults are more liable to develop severe paralysis in poliovirus infection than children: the risk of this is increased by pregnancy, tonsillectomy, fatigue, trauma or inoculation with bacterial vaccines.

Virology

1. Picornaviruses (pico = small + RNA)
2. RNA viruses, single-strand positive-sense RNA
3. Small, roughly spherical particles, 25–30 nm (Fig. 7.2)

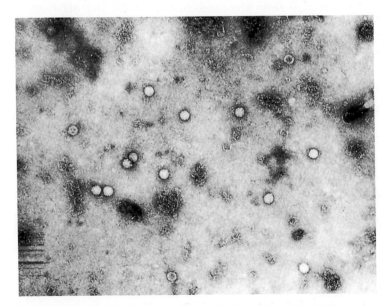

Fig. 7.2 Echovirus. All enteroviruses look like this, with very small virus particles with cubic symmetry. × 90 000. (Photograph by Dr E A C Follett.)

4. Stable at acid pH (hence survival in the intestinal tract)
5. Grow in tissue cultures with rapid CPE (except coxsackie A viruses)
6. Coxsackieviruses (but not polioviruses or echoviruses) are pathogenic for suckling mice.

Diagnosis

Isolation:

Specimens: faeces, throat swabs: CSF is useful for some viruses (e.g. echovirus 9) but not for polioviruses.

Inoculate: monkey kidney, human embryo lung cell cultures.

Observe: for CPE.

Type virus: by neutralization tests.

If coxsackie A virus infection is suspected:

Inoculate: suckling mice.

Observe: for signs of disease – group A coxsackieviruses cause flaccid paralysis due to myositis.

Note: Group B coxsackieviruses cause spastic paralysis in suckling mice, with tremor due to cerebral lesions and fat-pad necrosis.

Serology: not generally useful, with the following exceptions.

Neutralization tests: are sometimes used for the diagnosis of poliomyelitis (or the rare case of paralysis following vaccination).

ELISA test: to detect IgM to group B coxsackieviruses.

Direct demonstration: PCR is now available: used to detect enterovirus RNA in tissues and CSF.

Vaccination

Two vaccines are available against the three polioviruses.

Sabin live attenuated virus vaccine

Used for poliomyelitis immunization in the UK.

Contains: attenuated strains of the three polioviruses; grown in monkey kidney tissue culture.

Administration: in three oral doses along with triple vaccine at 2, 3 and 4 months old: boost at school entry and before leaving school.

Protection: good.

Blood antibody response: good.

Gut immunity: vaccinated children have resistance to alimentary infection, due to virus-specific IgA in the gut produced in response to the vaccine.

Safety: good; very rarely paralysis: usually mild and usually due to the type 3 component: incidence about one per million doses.

Vaccinated children are infectious to others, so vaccine strains may circulate to contacts in the community.

Contraindications: immunodeficient patients, pregnant women.

Widespread use of this vaccine has resulted in a dramatic decrease in paralytic poliomyelitis and in the elimination of wild poliovirus circulation in the community.

Salk inactivated virus vaccine

The first polio vaccine to be used on a large scale, but now less widely used than Sabin vaccine.

Contains: the three polioviruses, inactivated by formaldehyde.

Administration: in three subcutaneous injections.

Although producing good blood antibody levels – and therefore good protection against paralysis – it fails to give gut immunity. Nevertheless, modern Salk vaccine is of improved, high potency and is used successfully in Scandinavia.

Poliovirus eradication

The lack of an animal reservoir and the availability of effective vaccine make eradication of poliomyelitis a real possibility. This is now a priority aim for the World Health Organization and many continents are already 'poliovirus-free zones'. But note, some countries in Eastern Europe are still experiencing outbreaks of poliomyelitis and it is clear that wild viruses are continuing to circulate there.

8. Viral gastroenteritis

Viruses are an important cause of acute diarrhoea – most often, but not exclusively, in young children. In developing countries viral gastroenteritis plays a major role in the high infant mortality; in Britain the disease is now generally mild.

Several viruses are responsible: most do not grow in cell culture and were discovered – and are still often diagnosed – by electron microscopy.

The main viruses causing acute diarrhoea are listed in Table 8.1, which also indicates their particle morphology – an important method of differentiation.

Clinical features

Incubation period: short: 1–2 days.

Symptoms: acute onset of diarrhoea, often with vomiting – which may be projectile – and sometimes with fever: abdominal cramps are a characteristic feature: dehydration – with hyponatraemia – can be life-threatening in small children (Fig. 8.1).

Table 8.1 Viruses causing diarrhoea

Virus	Nucleic acid	Particle
Rotavirus	DS RNA in 11 segments	Double-shelled with wheel-like surface structure
Adenovirus	DS DNA	Classical icosahedron with rounded capsomeres
Astrovirus	SS RNA	Six-pointed star surface structure
SRSVs (Small, round, structured viruses)	SS RNA	Six-pointed star surface structure with central hole

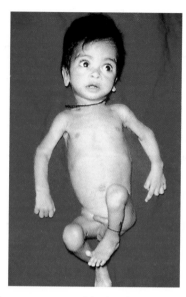

Fig. 8.1   Child with acute gastroenteritis, showing the characteristic appearance of dehydration. (Reproduced, with permission, from Abbott Laboratories 1982 Slide Atlas of Infectious Diseases. Gower Medical Publishing, London. Photograph by Professor H Lambert.)

Age: seen in all age groups (including the elderly), but more common in children.

Season: most common in the winter months.

Geographical distribution: world-wide distribution, but highest incidence in conditions of poor sanitation, overcrowding and poverty.

Epidemiology

Endemic infection: common in young children – especially group A rotaviruses and adenoviruses 40 and 41.

Epidemics or outbreaks of infection are seen, most often associated with SRSVs.

Treatment

Symptomatic: rehydration, with care to correct sodium loss (hyponatraemia) if rehydrating salt solutions are used too liberally.

ROTAVIRUS

The first virus found to cause acute non-bacterial gastroenteritis: mainly affects infants but outbreaks have been reported in adults – most often among the elderly, in hospitals or in residential homes.

Site of infection: upper small intestine.

Pathogenicity: there is no doubt that rotavirus causes diarrhoea, but infection is often symptomless – with virus found in the stools of healthy controls.

Transmission: faecal–oral from case to case, but respiratory symptoms have been described in rotavirus infection, raising the possibility that respiratory secretions may also be a source of spread.

Epidemiology

Infection is mainly endemic, but outbreaks – several in adults – have been reported.

Virology

1. Reovirus family.
2. RNA, double-stranded, 11 segments, which form characteristic banding patterns on electrophoresis (Fig. 8.2).

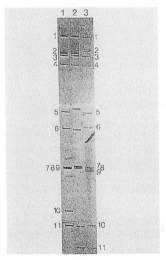

Fig. 8.2   The 11 RNA segments of the rotavirus genome can be separated by gel electrophoresis. The three rotavirus strains shown here are distinguishable by differences in the size – and so the migration into the gel – of their RNA segments. (Photograph by Dr U Desselberger.)

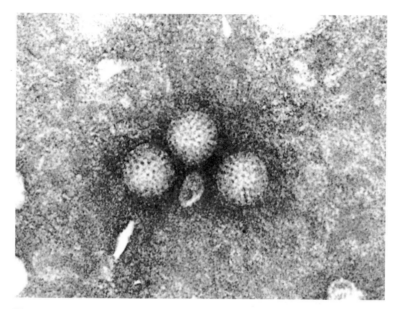

Fig. 8.3   Rotavirus. Spherical particles with cubic symmetry, showing characteristic outer layer like the spokes of a wheel, which distinguishes the virus from other reoviruses. × 200 000. (Photograph by Professor C R Madeley.)

3. Particles – are characteristic (Fig. 8.3 and Table 8.1).
4. Six groups are recognized, of which A, B and C contain the human pathogenic rotaviruses. Group A – the most common – contains several different serotypes.
5. Can now be grown in tissue culture, but only by special techniques.

Diagnosis

Demonstration of virus in the stools by electron microscopy.
Serology: (to detect antigen) ELISA, latex agglutination.

ADENOVIRUSES

Diarrhoea-causing adenoviruses (i.e. group F adenoviruses) are 'fastidious' in that they are cultivable only by specialized techniques: serologically distinct from respiratory strains. Found in endemic infections in the community and also in outbreaks: infection is often associated with prolonged excretion.

Virology

Faecal group F adenoviruses have the characteristic properties of all adenoviruses but belong to serotypes 40 and 41. Culture is not usually attempted in routine laboratories.

Diagnosis

Direct demonstration: by electron microscopy of stools.
 Serology: detection of antigen in stools by ELISA.

ASTROVIRUSES

Astroviruses cause diarrhoea mainly in children: they have been reported in several outbreaks in hospitals and within families.

Virology

1. RNA, single-stranded
2. Particles, distinguishable (but with difficulty) from those of SRSVs, which they resemble: see Table 8.1
3. Serotypes: five have been reported
4. Grow in tissue culture using special techniques.

Diagnosis

Direct demonstration: by electron microscopy of stools.

SMALL ROUND STRUCTURED VIRUSES (SRSVS)

Several animal species have their own caliciviruses. SRSVs are human caliciviruses, and an important cause of diarrhoea.

Clinical features

Incubation period: 24–48 h.
 Symptoms: abdominal cramps and vomiting are prominent features; low grade fever is present in about half the patients.
 Duration: lasts 48–72 h, usually without sequelae.
 Transmission: faecal–oral, but contamination of the environment with vomitus is also probably a route of infection: virus is excreted in the faeces for only up to 72 h.

Epidemiology

Outbreaks are common and have been reported associated with shellfish and water – and in hospitals and in residential homes for the elderly.

Virology

1. Caliciviruses
2. RNA viruses: single-strand positive-sense RNA
3. Electron microscopy (see Table 8.1)
4. Several types have been distinguished by genetic analysis of viral RNA
5. Do not grow in cell cultures.

Diagnosis

Direct demonstration:

Electron microscopy of stools.

PCR: to detect SRSV RNA in stools is now a practical method of diagnosis.

OTHER VIRUSES

Several other virus groups cause gastroenteritis in animals, and have been found in human stools: but their role in human disease is not proven.

These include:

- Toroviruses
- Enteroviruses
- Adenovirus serotypes (other than types 40 and 41).

9. Arthropod-borne virus infections

Many virus diseases are transmitted by the bite of an arthropod vector. The viruses are called *arboviruses*, and multiply in the bodies of the arthropods.

There are hundreds of arboviruses, many of which are not pathogenic for humans. They are classified into three main groups:

1. Alphavirus (formerly group A arboviruses)
2. Flavivirus (formerly group B arboviruses)
3. Bunyavirus.

Vectors: mosquitoes, ticks and sandflies are the principal arthropod vectors which transmit arboviruses.

Animal hosts: mainly wild birds and small mammals.

Transmission: via the bite of an insect vector, acquiring virus from a natural host and infecting humans by direct inoculation.

Geographical distribution: arboviruses are not a problem in Britain, where the only virus found is that causing the tick-borne disease *louping ill* in sheep – and very occasionally in humans.

Disease: arboviruses cause three types of disease:

1. Encephalitis
2. Fever – sometimes with rash
3. Haemorrhagic fever.

Note: these disease syndromes may overlap.

Some of the most important arboviruses are listed in Table 9.1, together with their vectors and the diseases they produce.

ARBOVIRUS ENCEPHALITIS

Arbovirus encephalitis is a world-wide problem. Found in:

1. **North and South America**: eastern and western equine encephalitis, rociovirus, California and St Louis encephalitis

Table 9.1   Some important arboviruses

Virus	Disease	Vector
Alphaviruses		
Eastern equine encephalitis	} Encephalitis	Mosquito
Western equine encephalitis		Mosquito
Venezuelan equine encephalitis	Encephalitis, fever	Mosquito
Chikungunya		Mosquito
Ross River	} Fever with polyarthritis	Mosquito
Mayava		Mosquito
Sindbis		Mosquito
Flaviviruses		
St Louis encephalitis	} Encephalitis	Mosquito
Japanese encephalitis		Mosquito
Murray Valley encephalitis		Mosquito
Tick-borne encephalitis		Tick
Rocio	Encephalitis	Mosquito
Yellow fever	Haemorrhagic fever	Mosquito
Kyasanur Forest disease	Haemorrhagic fever	Tick
Dengue	Fever, rash	Mosquito
West Nile fever	Haemorrhagic fever	Mosquito
Bunyaviruses		
California encephalitis	Encephalitis	Mosquito
Crimean-Congo haemorrhagic fever	Haemorrhagic fever	Tick
Rift Valley fever	Fever, haemorrhagic fever	Mosquito
Phlebotomus fever	Fever	Sandfly

2. *Far East*: Japanese encephalitis
3. *Europe*: tick-borne encephalitis
4. *Australia*: Murray Valley encephalitis.

Clinical features

Main symptoms: fever, progressively severe headache, nausea, vomiting, stiffness of neck, back and legs: progressing to convulsions, drowsiness, deepening coma and neurological signs such as paralysis and tremor.

Symptomless infection is common: after an epidemic, arbovirus antibodies are present in a considerable proportion of the population concerned, even though the incidence of encephalitis has been low. Some viruses, e.g. eastern equine encephalitis virus, cause CNS symptoms in a higher proportion of people infected than others, such as Venezuelan equine encephalitis virus.

Mortality: can be high: the case fatality rate varies but is highest with Japanese, eastern equine and Murray Valley encephalitis. In Europe, central European tick-borne encephalitis has a low case fatality rate (1–2%), whereas the similar virus of Far Eastern encephalitis has a case fatality rate of around 20%.

Neurological sequelae: often follow arbovirus encephalitis – again variable, depending on the virus involved: a particular problem in infants infected with Japanese and western and eastern equine encephalitis. Far Eastern encephalitis is commonly followed by residual flaccid paralysis of the arm and shoulder muscles.

Age: affects people of all ages, although some variations are seen with different viruses. For example, St Louis and eastern equine viruses are more likely to cause encephalitis when they infect the elderly. Western equine encephalitis, on the other hand, is more likely to cause symptomatic infection in infants.

Geographical distribution: arbovirus encephalitis is rare in most parts of Europe, with the exception of tick-borne or central European encephalitis: this disease is generally mild but its related virus, Far Eastern encephalitis (formerly called Russian spring-summer fever), is a severe disease.

Epidemiology

Epidemics in the countries affected are recurring and are seasonal – being more frequent in summer and in autumn.

Before and during a human epidemic there is a seasonal increase in the arthropod vector population – in most cases mosquitoes – with concomitant infection spreading in the animals that are the natural hosts of the virus: in eastern, western and Venezuelan equine encephalitis, epidemics of human infection are preceded by, or concurrent with, epidemic infection in horses – but horses, like humans, are secondary hosts of the viruses, the primary or natural hosts being birds.

ARBOVIRUS FEVERS AND HAEMORRHAGIC FEVERS

These syndromes overlap in that haemorrhages often complicate arbovirus fevers: some arboviruses cause arthritis and, with many, rash is a common feature.

Note: viral haemorrhagic fevers are also caused by other, non-arthropod-borne viruses (see Ch. 10).

Epidemiology

World-wide in distribution, but not seen in the UK and most other countries of Western Europe: distribution is related to vectors:

arbovirus fevers are therefore found mainly in semi-tropical and tropical countries where epidemics are a major health problem.

Clinical features

Symptomless infection – detected by a relatively high prevalence of antibodies in the general population concerned – is common.

Clinically, generalized febrile disease, which may be severe, with high fever, chills, sometimes headache, pain in the limbs, nausea and vomiting, rash: arthritis is seen with many arbovirus fevers and is typically a polyarthritis involving many joints.

Below, some of the best known arbovirus fevers are described.

Yellow fever

The most important arbovirus haemorrhagic fever, being the most severe, in which liver involvement and jaundice are prominent features. Historically, the cause of many deaths ('yellow jack') among early European colonialists settling in Central and South America. Still a problem despite an effective vaccine and its susceptibility to mosquito control measures. Endemic in South America and West Africa. There are two forms:

1. *Urban*: the reservoir of the virus is humans and the vector the mosquito *Aedes aegypti*.
2. *Sylvan or jungle*: the reservoir is tree-dwelling monkeys and the vector various species of forest mosquito.

Clinically, the most striking feature is jaundice due to viral involvement of the liver causing hepatitis; haemorrhages are common and toxic nephrosis with proteinuria a frequent complication.

Diagnosis: serology: by ELISA or haemagglutination-inhibition test.

Dengue

A major and growing health problem in many areas of the world, e.g. South East Asia, India, the Pacific islands, the Caribbean, where epidemics are recurring: humans are the main reservoir of infection and the main vector is *Aedes aegypti*.

Antigenic types: there are four subtypes (types 1 to 4) of dengue virus.

Clinically, dengue typically presents as a severe febrile disease with pain in the limbs and rash; the case fatality rate of this type of dengue is low.

Dengue haemorrhagic shock syndrome: a serious complication of dengue in young children. In this syndrome, an attack of dengue progresses to a more severe disease characterized by haemorrhages and shock: seen in children who have experienced a previous attack of dengue due to a different subtype of virus: antibody-mediated enhancement of infection is probably responsible for this, but the immunological mechanism involved is unclear.

Chikungunya

The cause of febrile disease with rash – sometimes in widespread epidemics – in Africa and Asia. In Asia the disease has had haemorrhagic manifestations.

Clinically, characterized by sudden fever with severe pain in the joints. Residual joint pains may persist after recovery from the acute disease.

O'nyong-nyong: due to a similar virus, febrile disease with joint pain (the name means 'break-bone fever'): seen in Africa in small outbreaks, but there was a large epidemic in 1959–60.

Ross River virus

The cause of epidemics in Australia and the Pacific of febrile disease with rash, in which polyarthritis is the predominant clinical feature.

Crimean-Congo haemorrhagic fever

A tick-borne bunyavirus disease seen over a large area, including the Middle East, the southern part of the former Soviet Union, Africa and the Far East: animal hosts include hares, ticks and birds: can also spread case-to-case to medical and nursing staff via contact with infected blood.

Clinically, the disease has a variable but sometimes high mortality: the most serious cases are marked by haemorrhages, sometimes with extensive skin ecchymoses and circulatory collapse.

Rift Valley fever

Responsible for large epizootics in sheep and cattle in Africa –

particularly Egypt, the Sudan and South Africa. Humans are infected through contact with infected animals or their tissues as well as via mosquito bite. The human disease is a febrile disease with headache, nausea, vomiting and haemorrhages in severe cases: some patients have developed retinitis.

ARBOVIRUSES

Virology

The following are some properties of arboviruses.

Alphaviruses

1. Some 37 recognized viruses, of which 13 cause disease in humans
2. RNA viruses: single-strand positive-sense RNA
3. Enveloped particles, roughly spherical, about 70 nm in diameter (Fig. 9.1)
4. Haemagglutinate avian red cells
5. Grow in cell culture: pathogenic for suckling mice.

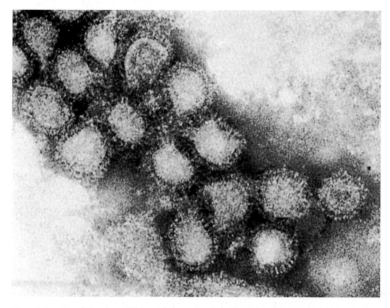

Fig. 9.1 An alphavirus. This photograph of sindbis virus shows roughly spherical particles with cubic symmetry and a surface fringe. × 200 000. (Photograph by Professor C R Madeley.)

Flaviviruses

1. More than 70 viruses
2. RNA viruses: single-strand positive-sense RNA
3. Enveloped particles: from 40–50 nm in diameter
4. Haemagglutinate avian red cells
5. Grow in cell culture: pathogenic for suckling mice.

Bunyaviruses

1. A large family containing nearly 300 viruses
2. RNA viruses: single-strand negative-sense RNA in three segments
3. Enveloped particles, approximately 90–100 nm in diameter
4. Haemagglutinate
5. Grow in cell culture: generally pathogenic for suckling mice or other rodents.

Diagnosis of arbovirus infection

Generally requires facilities of specialist reference laboratories.
   Serology:
   Haemagglutination-inhibition for rising titres.
   ELISA for IgM detection.
   Isolation:
   Specimens: blood (sometimes throat swab, CSF, etc.).
   Inoculate: suckling mice; cell culture (where appropriate); mosquito larvae.

Vaccines

The most widely used vaccine available for arboviruses is against yellow fever – but effective vaccines are also available for Japanese and tick-borne encephalitis, and on a limited basis, for those at special risk, for eastern and western equine encephalitis. Research into a vaccine for dengue is ongoing.

Yellow fever vaccine

Contains: live attenuated virus of a strain known as 17D, attenuated by repeated passage in chick embryos.
   Prepared: in chick embryos.

Administration: in one dose by subcutaneous injection.

Protection conferred: is good, solid immunity which lasts for at least 10 years.

Safety: good: singularly free from side-effects.

Japanese encephalitis vaccine

Recommended for travellers to endemic areas in South East Asia and the Far East.

Contains: inactivated virus.

Prepared: in mouse brain.

Administration: in three doses subcutaneously.

In the UK: unlicensed but available on a named-patient basis.

Tick-borne encephalitis vaccine

Recommended for travellers (especially walkers and campers) in endemic areas in Scandinavia, and in central and Eastern Europe.

Contains: inactivated virus.

Prepared: in chick embryo cells.

Administration: in two doses intramuscularly, 4–12 weeks apart.

10. Rabies; non-arthropod-borne haemorrhagic fevers

The diseases to be described in this chapter are *zoonoses*, i.e. they are acquired from animals which are reservoirs of infection.

RABIES

Rabies is a lethal form of encephalitis due to a virus which affects a wide variety of animal species: rabies is transmitted to humans via the bite of an infected animal which is usually – but not always – a dog.

Clinical features

Incubation period: long: usually 4–12 weeks, sometimes much longer; if the bite is on the head or neck the incubation period is shorter than for bites on the limbs. Virus spread from the wound to the CNS is via the nerves.

Symptoms: initially: nonspecific, often early psychological symptoms such as personality changes, apprehension, etc.: paraesthesia around the wound is another early symptom. Thereafter there are two forms of rabies:

1. *Furious*: the more common: symptoms are excitement, with tremor, muscular contractions and convulsions; typically, spasm of the muscles of swallowing (hence the older name for the disease of 'hydrophobia' or fear of water) and increased sensitivity of the sensory nervous system (Fig. 10.1).

2. *Dumb or paralytic* rabies: symptoms of ascending paralysis, eventually involving the muscles of swallowing, speech and respiration.

Virus is present in saliva, skin and eyes as well as the brain.

Prognosis: the disease is virtually always fatal (although there

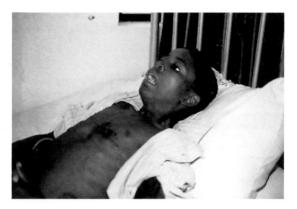

Fig. 10.1   Rabies. Patient in hydrophobic spasm. (Photograph by Dr D A Warrell.)

have been rare reports of recovery); death often follows a convulsion.

Pathology: despite the severity of the clinical disease, lesions in the CNS are often minimal, with little evidence of destructive effects on cells, but with intracytoplasmic inclusions within neurones known as *Negri bodies*, which are diagnostic of rabies.

Epidemiology

Rabies infects dogs, cats, bats and carnivorous wild animals such as foxes (Europe), wolves (former Soviet Union), and skunks (USA); in these animal populations the virus is enzootic. Infection is also found in rodents and cattle (especially in South America, where the virus is spread by the bite of infected vampire bats).

Dogs are the main danger to humans: virus is present in the saliva of infected dogs – for up to 7 days (but rarely for more than 4 days) before the onset of symptoms of the disease; dogs and cats which remain healthy for 10 days after biting can be regarded as being free of virus at the time of biting.

Incidence of rabies after biting: most dog bites are, of course, from non-rabid animals: only about 15% of people bitten by a rabid animal develop the disease; bites on the head or neck carry a greater risk of rabies than those on the limbs. Post-exposure vaccination now offers effective prophylaxis against rabies.

Britain is free from indigenous rabies. Rabies used to be present in animals in Britain, but was eradicated by 1921; the strict 6-month quarantine laws for imported animals have been successful in keeping out the disease: but this policy is now being reconsidered. Smuggling of pet animals into Britain has in the past caused importation of the virus into the country. The main danger is that rabies might become established as a reservoir of infection in wild animals – and Britain has a large fox population.

Wild animals: rabies is present in wild animals in all continents of the world, with the exception of Australia and Antarctica. Rabies has been spreading in Europe as an epizootic in foxes since 1945, slowly moving westward from Eastern Europe to France over the past 50 years or so: however this epizootic has been controlled by effective wildlife vaccination programmes.

Bats: lyssaviruses, related to rabies virus, are presently epizootic in European bats; although less dangerous to humans than rabies, occasional cases of human infection have been attributed to them.

Aerosol infection: has been recorded – as a result of laboratory accident, or by exposure in bat-infested caves: a rare event.

Case-to-case spread: human patients do not seem to be infectious to medical attendants, despite the presence of virus in saliva: nevertheless, vaccination is advisable.

Corneal transplant: cases of rabies in recipients of corneas from donors with undiagnosed rabies have been reported.

Virology

1. A lyssavirus within the rhabdovirus family: rabies is the most neurotropic of the antigenically-related lyssaviruses which infect many different animal species. Sporadic cases of rabies-like disease have been due to other lyssaviruses, infecting bats and other animals such as shrews.

2. RNA virus: single-strand negative-sense RNA.

3. Bullet-shaped, enveloped particles containing helically-coiled nucleoprotein: length 180 nm, diameter 70–80 nm (Fig. 10.2).

4. Haemagglutinates goose erythrocytes.

5. Grows – but poorly – in a line of murine neuroblastoma cells with eosinophilic cytoplasmic inclusions, but usually without CPE.

6. Pathogenic for mice and other laboratory animals.

Diagnosis

Direct demonstration of virus:

Specimens: hair-bearing skin (e.g. back of neck), corneal impression smears, brain tissue.

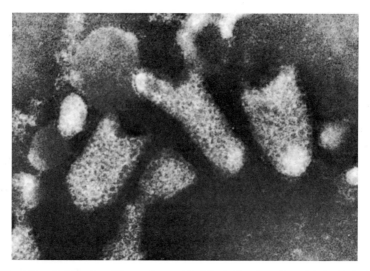

Fig. 10.2   Rabies virus. The nucleocapsid of the bullet-shaped particle has helical symmetry and is surrounded by an envelope. × 180 000. (Photograph by Professor C R Madeley.)

Examine: for presence of rabies virus antigen by immuno-fluorescence.

Isolation:

Specimens: brain tissue, saliva, CSF, urine.

Inoculate: mice intracerebrally.

Observe: for paralysis, convulsions; post-mortem for immuno-fluorescence with rabies antiserum and Negri bodies in brain cells.

Note: rabies is difficult to diagnose during life. Specimens are often negative and serological results difficult to interpret if immunization has been undertaken. RNA detection by PCR (see Ch. 3) now offers a sensitive and reliable method of confirming the diagnosis in the laboratory.

Post-mortem

Negri bodies: examine brain smears of the Ammon's horn of the hippocampus by immunofluorescence with rabies antiserum and, for Negri bodies, with Seller's stain for red intracytoplasmic inclusions.

Dogs

If rabies is suspected, the dog should be kept under observation to see if the disease develops; if killed before death due to the disease, Negri bodies may not have developed in sufficient numbers to be detected in histological sections. After death, the dog's head is sent to a specialist laboratory for examination.

Vaccination

The long incubation period makes rabies a suitable disease for prophylactic immunization after exposure.

Rabies vaccine was first developed by Pasteur in 1885; it consisted of virus attenuated by drying the spinal cords of infected rabbits for varying lengths of time, over KOH. Wild rabies virus is known as *street* virus and attenuated virus as *fixed* virus. Allergic encephalomyelitis was a not infrequent complication of vaccines – like Pasteur's – which had been prepared in animal nervous tissue. All vaccines prepared for human use contain inactivated virus.

After exposure – or suspicion of exposure – to rabies, the wound should be thoroughly washed with soap and water, alcohol, iodine solutions or a quaternary ammonium compound. Patients should be given combined passive and active immunization:

- Passive immunization: by injection of human anti-rabies immunoglobulin
- Active immunization: should be started immediately after passive immunization.

Human diploid cell vaccine

The main vaccine in use is human diploid cell vaccine (HDCV) – now the vaccine of choice.

Contains: inactivated virus.

Prepared: in human diploid embryo lung cells.

Administration: intramuscularly or subcutaneously into the deltoid area of the upper arm, in five doses spaced at 0, 3, 7, 14 and 30 days.

Protection: effective: produces high levels of neutralizing antibody.

Safety: good: some local reaction is not uncommon.

Animal vaccines

Contain: inactivated virus.

Used: for dogs – an important control measure: also available for cats and cattle in endemic areas, and occasionally other animals:

for example, those in zoos, or particularly valuable stock, should be vaccinated.

Wild animals: trials in Europe of live attenuated virus vaccine distributed in bait have proved successful in eradicating rabies in wildlife; this might in time lead to the eradication of the disease.

Pre-exposure vaccination

Veterinary surgeons, animal handlers, laboratory workers or others at high risk from rabies should be given three doses of vaccine at 0, 7 and 28 days, with boosters every 2–3 years. Two booster doses should be given if they are bitten or otherwise exposed to infection.

MARBURG AND EBOLA VIRUS DISEASES

Marburg is a severe disease which first appeared in 1967 in an outbreak initially involving laboratory workers in Marburg, Frankfurt and Belgrade, who had handled the tissues from a batch of African green monkeys. Later, there were other cases in contacts of the patients. The monkeys may have been infected during transit. Ebola – an equally or even more severe disease – has appeared in outbreaks in Sudan and West Africa.

Clinical features

Clinically, both diseases are very severe febrile illnesses with headache, myalgia, maculopapular rash and haemorrhagic manifestations; other features are vomiting, diarrhoea, hepatitis, pharyngitis and signs of renal and CNS involvement. There is leucopenia, with atypical lymphocytes and plasma cells in the blood and signs of vascular damage.

Case fatality rate is high – considerably more than 50% in the Ebola outbreaks.

Infectiousness: a feature of both diseases is the ability to spread directly from case to case: several of the infections have been in medical attendants of patients with the disease.

Epidemiology

Marburg disease appeared again in 1975 in two young people in South Africa. In 1976 there were outbreaks of Ebola infection, with many deaths in Sudan and Zaire, and in 1995 there was another severe outbreak in Zaire. Ebola virus was identified in monkeys imported from the Philippines to the USA in 1989–90, showing that the virus was present outside Africa, although this virus appeared to be less pathogenic than the viruses isolated in earlier human outbreaks. The host species of both Marburg and Ebola viruses are unknown, although it seems likely that monkeys are involved.

Virology

1. Filoviruses: two serologically distinct viruses: Marburg and Ebola
2. RNA viruses
3. Unusual particles: long, branching, filamentous, with hooked ends. Variable length, diameter 80 nm: enveloped with surface projections
4. Grow in various tissue cultures, without CPE but with intracytoplasmic inclusions
5. Pathogenic for guinea-pigs.

Diagnosis

Isolation:

Specimen: blood.

Inoculate: guinea-pigs (intraperitoneally) or cell cultures.

Observe: guinea-pigs for signs of febrile illness, with detection of virus antigen by immunofluorescence in lesions in liver, lymph nodes or spleen; or *cell cultures* for intracytoplasmic inclusions and by immunofluorescence.

Serology: indirect immunofluorescence.

ARENAVIRUSES

There are three main human pathogenic arenaviruses or arena-virus groups:

1. Lassa fever virus
2. The Tacaribe complex of viruses associated with South American arenaviruses
3. Lymphocytic choriomeningitis.

The natural hosts of all the viruses are mice or rats.

Transmission: infection is acquired by inhalation or ingestion of materials contaminated with rodent excreta, or direct contamination of cuts, etc. Lassa fever can also be acquired by direct contact with a case of the disease.

Virology

1. RNA viruses: the genome is contained in two RNA segments
2. Medium-sized, 110 nm enveloped particles with internal granules which are host cell ribosomes
3. Grow in Vero cells
4. Pathogenic for mice and guinea-pigs.

LASSA FEVER

A febrile disease endemic in West Africa, which was first reported in Lassa, Nigeria. The virus can be highly infectious and can spread to medical and nursing personnel looking after patients. The multi-mammate rat is the reservoir of the virus.

Clinical features

The illness starts with fever and sore throat: then vomiting, cough, weakness and malaise, ulcers in the mouth and pharynx and cervical lymphadenopathy; facial oedema is a prominent sign; abdominal pain, myalgia with diarrhoea; encephalopathy with headache is common; late features are haemorrhage and shock: deafness is also a late complication.

Case fatality is overall 2%, although it is higher (16%) in hospitalized patients. Not all cases are severe – many infections are mild.

Symptomless infection: is common within rural populations.

Diagnosis

Serology: by immunofluorescence or ELISA.

Note: in the UK the diagnosis may be missed unless a history of recent travel to West Africa is sought. Patients in hospital wards need to be nursed in isolation facilities, as they can represent an infectious hazard to staff.

Treatment

Ribavirin: effective if given early.

SOUTH AMERICAN HAEMORRHAGIC FEVERS

These are due to four related arenaviruses, which together form the Tacaribe complex:

1. *Junin*: Argentina
2. *Machupo*: Bolivia
3. *Guanarito*: Venezuela
4. *Sabia*: Brazil.

Clinically: severe diseases with haemorrhagic, renal, cardiovascular and sometimes neurological symptoms. The reservoirs of the viruses are rats or mouse-like rodents.

The Argentinian disease is rural and spreads mainly during the maize harvest from mice which inhabit the maize fields: there have been large and severe annual outbreaks of the disease amongst the corn harvesters there, although vaccination may be helping to control these.

The Bolivian disease was mostly acquired in houses and is now rare.

Guanarito and Sabia viruses have caused outbreaks of severe disease in Venezuela and Brazil respectively.

Vaccine

An attenuated Junin virus vaccine has been developed for use in at-risk populations in Argentina.

LYMPHOCYTIC CHORIOMENINGITIS

A widespread natural infection in mice: the virus is excreted in the urine and faeces of infected mice; transmission to humans appears to be a rare event. The disease has also been acquired from pet and laboratory hamsters.

The disease is of interest from an immunological point of view, since mice are not uncommonly infected in utero; when this happens they have a generalized infection with high titres of virus in all tissues and organs: however, the mice remain symptomless –

although they later succumb to glomerulonephritis due to immune complex deposition in the kidney.

Clinical features

The most important syndrome in humans is aseptic meningitis; sometimes meningoencephalitis is seen; the virus also causes an influenza-like febrile illness.

HANTAVIRUSES

Hantaviruses are rodent viruses which can spread to humans. Rodent infection is chronic and symptomless, but in humans these viruses can cause severe febrile illness: they belong to the bunyavirus family.

Clinical features

Three main syndromes are seen:

1. *Haemorrhagic fever with renal syndrome*: a severe disease with fever, renal impairment including proteinuria and oliguria, and haemorrhages: abdominal pain is common. Recovery is slow with prolonged convalescence, and the mortality is around 5%.

2. *Nephropathia epidemica*: a milder febrile illness with prominent signs of renal dysfunction. Around half the patients have abdominal pain.

3. *Hantavirus pulmonary syndrome*: a very severe disease with a high case fatality rate – around 50%: a febrile illness with severe respiratory failure and cardiogenic shock: gross pleural effusions are seen in some patients.

Four main virus-specific syndromes are seen:

1. *Hantaan virus*: found in Korea, Eastern Russia, China (associated with rats): causes haemorrhagic fever with renal syndrome

2. *Puumala virus*: endemic in bank voles (and probably also in other rodents) in Scandinavia and Western Europe: causes nephropathia epidemica

3. *Sin nombre (no name) virus*: the cause of hantavirus pulmonary syndrome and of which the natural host is the deer mouse: found mainly in the western USA

4. *Seoul virus*: is widespread in rats world-wide, but seems rarely to cause disease in humans.

Epidemiology

Transmission: mainly air-borne, but arthropod vectors (such as rodent mites) may play a role. Infection has been reported in laboratory workers, presumably from handling experimental rodents. No human-to-human transmission has been recorded.

Geographical distribution: different hantaviruses tend to be associated with specific rodent hosts, and are found in certain parts of the world depending on the geographical distribution of their rodent host.

Virology

1. Members of bunyavirus family
2. Single-stranded RNA in three segments
3. Enveloped particles with surface projections; many with internal granules
4. Grow, but with great difficulty, in cell culture.

Diagnosis

Serology: by immunofluorescence or ELISA.

Treatment

Ribavirin has been used intravenously to treat severe infection, but is of uncertain value.

11. Herpesvirus diseases

Most animal species, including humans, are hosts for a particular herpesvirus, and sometimes for two or more. All herpesviruses are morphologically identical and have the important property of remaining latent, in potentially viable form, within the cells of the host after primary infection. Latent virus persists for long periods of time – probably throughout life: some herpesviruses reactivate from time to time from the latent state, to produce recurrent infection.

There are eight recognized human herpesviruses:

1. Herpes simplex virus type 1
2. Herpes simplex virus type 2
3. Varicella-zoster virus
4. Cytomegalovirus
5. Epstein-Barr (EB) virus
6. Human herpesvirus 6
7. Human herpesvirus 7
8. Human herpesvirus 8.

HERPES SIMPLEX VIRUS

Herpes simplex virus is unusual among viruses in causing a wide variety of clinical syndromes: the basic lesions are vesicles, but these can take many different forms.

There are two types of herpes simplex virus:

- Type 1: the commonest: causes mainly oro-facial lesions
- Type 2: the main cause of genital herpes.

Diseases due to the virus fall into two categories:

1. Primary: when the virus is first encountered
2. Reactivation: recurrent infections, due to reactivation of latent virus.

93

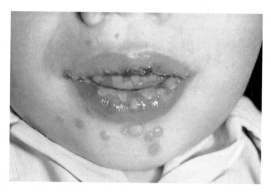

Fig. 11.1   Primary herpes simplex infection. Stomatitis with satellite vesicles over the chin. (Reproduced, with permission, from Grist N R, Ho-Yen D O, Walker E, Williams G R 1988 Diseases of infection. Oxford University Press.)

Primary infections

Most primary infections are symptomless. Below are listed the main clinical manifestations when primary infection is symptomatic.

Gingivostomatitis

Vesicles inside the mouth on the buccal mucosa and on the gums: these ulcerate and become coated with a greyish slough (Fig. 11.1): the commonest primary disease, because kissing is the main route of virus spread, but vesicles may be produced at other sites, most often on the head or neck.

Herpetic whitlow

Due to implantation of the virus into the fingers: the lesion produced looks very similar to a staphylococcal whitlow, but the exudate is serous rather than purulent: an occupational hazard of doctors and nurses, especially of anaesthetists or neurosurgical nurses, who deal with unconscious patients who are intubated: infection is acquired through contamination of the hands by virus in saliva or respiratory secretions.

Conjunctivitis and keratitis

Primary herpes can involve the eye – both conjunctiva and cornea: the eyelids are generally swollen and there are often vesicles and ulcers on them.

Kaposi's varicelliform eruption

This is a superinfection of eczematous skin: mainly seen in young children; sometimes a serious disease with a significant fatality rate.

Acute necrotizing encephalitis

A rare but severe disease: clinically, presents with the sudden onset of fever, mental confusion and headache: the main site of infection is the temporal lobe, where the disease causes necrosis. Recently a milder form of herpes encephalitis, with a better prognosis, has been described – usually in children. It is uncertain whether herpes encephalitis is a primary infection or a reactivation.

Genital herpes

A vesicular eruption of the genital area, most often due to herpes simplex virus type 2: sexually transmitted; due to type 1 virus in a quarter to a third of cases.

Neonatal infection

Severe generalized infection in neonates is usually acquired from a primary genital infection in the mother, when no maternal antibody is present for the protection of the child. Affected infants have jaundice, hepatosplenomegaly, thrombocytopenia and large vesicular lesions on the skin: there is a high case fatality rate: usually due to herpes simplex virus type 2 (unless acquired from a nurse or other person in the maternity ward who is suffering from a type 1 lesion).

Generalized infection in adults

This is a rare manifestation of primary infection with type 1 virus, with disseminated vesicular skin lesions and virus in viscera and other body organs and tissues: *herpes hepatitis* has also been described.

Latency

During primary infection, the virus travels via sensory nerves from the site of infection in the mouth to the trigeminal ganglion – and other cranial and cervical ganglia also. Virus remains in ganglia in a potentially viable state, and in a proportion of people reactivates to cause recurrent infection. Virus can be isolated from the trigeminal ganglia of people who suffer reactivation – and from some who do not. In genital herpes, type 2 becomes latent in the sacral ganglia.

Clinical reactivation

Reactivation of virus is provoked by stimuli, such as common colds, sunlight (possibly a result of exposure to ultraviolet light), pneumonia, stress, menstruation. Reactivation recurs sporadically, sometimes often, throughout life.

Neutralizing antibody is produced after primary infection, but does not prevent reactivation: virus is protected from serum antibody within the axons of sensory nerves as it travels to the site of recurrent infection. Reactivation does not stimulate a rise in titre of herpes antibody.

Cold sores

Vesicles at mucocutaneous junctions of nose and mouth are the most common manifestation (Fig. 11.2): these progress to pustules with crust formation: the virus travels from the trigeminal ganglion down the maxillary or mandibular branches of the trigeminal nerve to reach areas of the skin supplied by these nerves. Herpetic

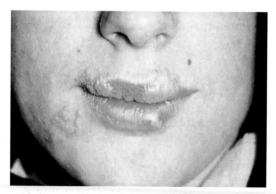

Fig. 11.2   Vesicular cold sores – the commonest disease due to herpes simplex virus. The virus has reactivated from the latent state in the trigeminal ganglion. (Reproduced, with permission, from Topley and Wilson's Principles of Bacteriology, Virology and Immunity, 8th edn 1990. Edward Arnold, London, vol 4.)

vesicles can recur – but more rarely – at other sites on the skin: genital lesions also recur, most often with type 2 virus: less often when the primary genital lesions are due to type 1 virus.

Dendritic ulcer of the cornea

Reactivation less often affects the eye: recurrent lesions are – at least at first – restricted to the cornea: virus reaches the cornea via the ophthalmic branch of the trigeminal nerve. Lesions take the form of a branching or dendritic ulcer – a form of keratitis (Fig. 11.3): if recurrence is frequent, scarring develops and the disease may progress to a severe, destructive uveitis.

Immunosuppressive therapy

Patients with organ transplants may develop severe, extensive cold sores: usually in the mouth, these can become necrotic and spread onto the face and into the oesophagus. This is due to deficient cell-mediated immunity: but most transplant patients have the usual, self-limiting herpes reactivations.

Epidemiology

Prevalence: infection is virtually universal in human populations, and in elderly people the prevalence of antibody (indicating previous infection) is almost 100%.

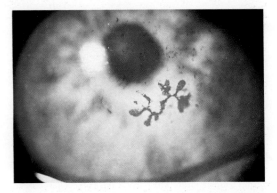

Fig. 11.3   Dendritic (branching) ulcer of the cornea, stained with rose bengal – another disease due to recurrent herpes simplex. (Photograph by Professor W R Lee, University of Glasgow.)

Transmission: by close personal contact, e.g. kissing (type 1 virus), sexual intercourse (type 2 virus).

Sources: generally people with herpetic lesions; however, carriers of latent virus from time to time secrete virus in their saliva without any symptoms, and this may act as a source of (undetected) infection.

Age: infection is most common in childhood and is usually symptomless: there is another peak in incidence during adolescence, due to kissing as contact with the opposite gender increases.

Virology

1. Roughly spherical enveloped particle with characteristic morphology, 100 nm (Fig. 11.4)
2. Double-stranded DNA
3. Types 1 and 2 share group-specific antigens, but can be differentiated by type-specific antigens and by DNA restriction enzyme analysis

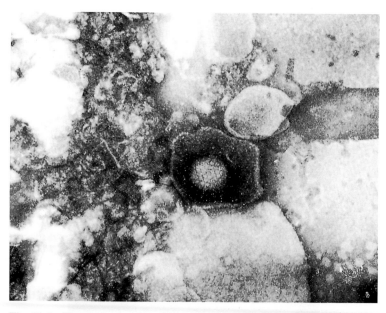

Fig. 11.4 Herpes simplex virus. The particle has cubic symmetry and the capsid is composed of hollow-cored capsomeres. There is a loose, baggy envelope. × 108 000. (Photograph by Dr E A C Follett.)

4. Grows in most cell cultures, with characteristic CPE with ballooning and rounding of cells
5. Pathogenic in laboratory animals, causing encephalitis.

Diagnosis

Isolation:

Specimens: swab or fluid from vesicles, skin, saliva, conjunctiva; corneal scrapings, brain biopsy.

Inoculate: cell cultures.

Observe: for CPE of rounded cells.

Type virus: by immunofluorescence or neutralization.

Serology:

Complement fixation test: useful for diagnosing primary infections; difficult to interpret in recurrent infections because of existing antibody and because recurrences do not usually cause a rise in titre.

Direct demonstration: of virus or virus antigen in vesicles or other fluids or tissues, by electron microscopy or immunofluorescence.

Herpes encephalitis: PCR is now used to detect herpes-specific DNA in CSF in cases of suspected encephalitis: can also be diagnosed by demonstration of antibody locally produced in CSF, i.e. by increase in normal CSF/serum antibody ratio.

Treatment

(See also Chapter 18.)

Acyclovir

Treatment of herpes simplex has been revolutionized by the introduction of this non-toxic drug which has a specific inhibitory action on herpes simplex virus replication.

Administration: intravenously, orally or topically.

Indications: herpes encephalitis, severe or generalized herpes (given systemically); genital herpes (systemically or orally); dendritic ulcers, cold sores, possibly genital herpes (topically); prophylaxis in immunocompromised patients.

Also used: valaciclovir (a prodrug of acyclovir) and famciclovir (recommended for genital herpes).

VARICELLA-ZOSTER VIRUS

Varicella (chickenpox) and zoster (shingles – but also sometimes called 'herpes zoster') are different diseases due to the same virus:

- **Varicella** is the primary illness
- **Zoster** is a reactivation of infection.

Varicella

Clinical features

Incubation period: 10–21 days.

One of the common childhood fevers: a mild febrile illness with a characteristic vesicular rash: vesicles appear in successive waves so that lesions of different ages are present together: the vesicles (in which there are giant cells) develop into pustules; virus is shed – in respiratory secretions – from 48 h before the rash appears and is also present in the vesicular lesions.

Complications are rare: post-infectious encephalitis, haemorrhagic (fulminating) varicella; in adults, pneumonia is a relatively common and serious complication and may be followed by pulmonary calcification: pulmonary involvement is dangerous in pregnancy and may cause serious disease and occasionally death.

Congenital varicella: rare: maternal varicella in early pregnancy is occasionally followed, in the infant, by a syndrome of limb hypoplasia, muscular atrophy and cerebral and psychomotor retardation.

Perinatal or neonatal varicella: maternal varicella near the time of delivery may also affect the child. If the mother contracts varicella more than 7 days before delivery, the disease in the child is usually mild: this is because the child's disease is modified by placentally transmitted early maternal antibody; within 7 days of delivery, there is no maternal antibody and the child is liable to develop severe disease.

Pregnancy: varicella can be unusually severe in pregnant women.

Immunity: attack is followed by solid and long-lasting immunity to varicella – but *not to zoster*.

Epidemiology

Seasonal distribution: highest incidence is in late winter and early spring.

Transmission: via inhalation of respiratory secretions, or via virus present in skin lesions.

Varicella (cf. zoster) is an epidemic disease; acquired by contact with cases of varicella or (less commonly) of zoster.

Zoster

Clinical features

A reactivation of virus latent in dorsal root or cranial nerve ganglia following – and usually many years after – childhood varicella. Virus travels down sensory nerves to produce painful vesicles in the area of skin (dermatome) innervated from the affected ganglion.

Virus: is present in the skin vesicles and in the ganglia involved (where there are cytopathic changes of cell destruction and marked inflammatory infiltration).

Age: incidence rises with age: zoster is much more common in the elderly.

Ganglia: dorsal root ganglia – and therefore the thoracic nerves supplying dermatomes of the chest wall – are most often affected: there is a segmental rash which extends from the middle of the back in a horizontal strip round the side of the chest – 'a belt of roses from hell' (Fig. 11.5).

Cranial zoster: reactivation in the trigeminal ganglion involving the ophthalmic nerve causes a sharply demarcated area of lesions down one side of the forehead and scalp: in about half the patients, there are lesions in the eye.

Ramsay Hunt's syndrome is a rare form of zoster: the eruption is on the tympanic membrane and the external auditory canal and there is often a facial nerve palsy and sometimes loss of

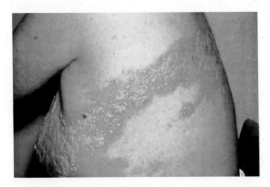

Fig. 11.5   Zoster. Thoracic rash with characteristic distribution of lesions, 'a belt of roses from hell'. (Photograph by Dr Alan Lyell.)

taste on the anterior two-thirds of the tongue: zoster has also been implicated in Bell's palsy.

Residual neuralgia – which may be severe – often follows zoster in the elderly.

Neurological signs are sometimes seen, e.g. paralysis.

Epidemiology

Cases are sporadic: there is no seasonal distribution.

Zoster – unlike varicella – is not acquired by contact with cases of either varicella or zoster – although it may give rise to varicella in susceptible contacts.

Virology

1. Double-stranded DNA virus with typical herpes particle morphology
2. Grows slowly in tissue cultures of human cells (e.g. human embryo lung), with focal CPE.

Diagnosis

Serology:

ELISA for IgM or *complement fixation test*: often useful for both varicella and zoster: unlike reactivations of herpes simplex, zoster usually causes a rise in antibody titre.

Rapid latex test: for detection of antibody indicating pre-existing immunity.

Direct demonstration: of herpesvirus particles in vesicle fluid by electron microscopy is a quick method of confirming a clinical diagnosis (but note, this does not distinguish varicella-zoster from herpes simplex virus).

Isolation: but grows only slowly in human embryo lung cells.

Treatment

(See also Chapter 18.)

Acyclovir

Severe varicella or zoster (e.g. in the immunocompromised) responds well: the virus is less sensitive than herpes simplex, but low toxicity means that dosage can be increased to produce inhibitory levels of the drug in blood and tissues.

Famciclovir

Similar in action to acyclovir, but can be given less often and in lower dosage.

Prophylaxis

Varicella-zoster immunoglobulin (ZIG)

Prepared from pooled plasma with high titres of varicella-zoster antibody: useful for prophylaxis or for reducing the severity of varicella in vulnerable contacts of varicella or (less often) zoster, including:

- Children or adults who are immunosuppressed because of disease or therapy (e.g. with organ transplants)
- Neonates born to mothers who contract varicella less than 7 days before or within 28 days after delivery
- Non-immune neonates exposed to varicella during the first 28 days after birth
- Non-immune pregnant women exposed to varicella.

Administration: intramuscularly, not more than 10 days after exposure.

Protection: not complete: about half those exposed to varicella and given ZIG develop varicella, but the disease is usually mild – i.e. ZIG has an ameliorating effect.

Vaccine

A live attenuated virus vaccine has been prepared but is not licensed in the UK: nevertheless it can be prescribed on a named patient basis: mainly used for children with leukaemia or solid tumours, and provides apparently good protection.

CYTOMEGALOVIRUS

Infection in the previously healthy is generally – but not always – symptomless: but like rubella, cytomegalovirus can infect the fetus during maternal infection in pregnancy. Now a major problem in transplant patients.

Most adults have antibody to the virus, showing that infection is widespread and common.

Latency: the virus is known to reactivate from the latent state, probably in polymorphonuclear leucocytes or lymphocytes but perhaps in other organs and cell types also.

There are two types of disease due to cytomegalovirus:

- Congenital
- Postnatal.

Congenital disease

A more difficult problem than congenital rubella because:

1. maternal infection is almost always symptomless
2. the fetus can be damaged by infection in any of the three trimesters of pregnancy
3. fetal infection can follow reactivation as well as primary maternal infection
4. approximately 0.4% of British children are congenitally infected, but most do not suffer sequelae (termination therefore presents ethical problems).

Clinical features

The majority of congenitally infected neonates show no signs or symptoms, and diagnosis is made by virological tests. Many of the children develop normally, although some show neurological sequelae later in life, principally deafness and/or mental retardation.

About 7% of infected infants develop severe generalized (or cytomegalic inclusion) disease.

Signs and symptoms: jaundice, hepatosplenomegaly, blood dyscrasias such as thrombocytopenia and haemolytic anaemia; the brain is almost always involved and some infants have micro-cephaly: motor disorders are common; surviving infants are usually deaf and mentally retarded. Cytomegalovirus probably causes about 10% of cases of microcephaly.

Affected organs: show characteristically enlarged cells (hence the prefix 'cytomegalo') with large intranuclear 'owl's eye' inclusions.

Postnatal disease

Hepatitis

In young children, primary infection with cytomegalovirus can – although rarely – cause hepatitis with enlargement of the liver and disturbance of liver function tests; jaundice may or may not be present.

Infectious mononucleosis syndrome

In adults and in older children, infection can give rise to infectious mononucleosis (see below), but with a negative Paul-Bunnell reaction and no lymphadenopathy or pharyngitis. There is fever, hepatitis and lymphocytosis, with atypical lymphocytes in the peripheral blood; sometimes seen after transfusion with fresh unfrozen blood or platelets – screening of donors for cytomegalovirus is now carried out to prevent this, and also to prevent infection being transmitted to recipients of transplants.

Infection in the immunocompromised

Disseminated infection is sometimes seen in immunodeficient patients, with widespread lesions in lungs as well as other organs and tissues, e.g. adrenals, liver and alimentary tract: a major complication of transplantation surgery.

Transplant patients are subject to frequent infections with cytomegalovirus – sometimes reactivations, sometimes due to infection acquired from the donor organ: not infrequently symptomless with renal transplants, but a major problem with bone marrow and heart transplant patients.

Pneumonia and retinitis are the main diseases associated with cytomegalovirus in transplant patients. Cytomegalovirus retinitis is a particular problem in AIDS patients (Fig. 11.6).

Virology

1. Double-stranded DNA
2. Grows slowly in cultures of human embryo lung cells, with characteristic focal CPE.

Diagnosis

***Isolation*:**
Specimens: urine, throat gargle, blood (non-coagulated).
Inoculate: human embryo lung cell cultures.
Observe: the direct early antigen fluorescent foci test (DEAFF) is a rapid method of detecting early virus growth in cell culture at 24 or 48 h: CPE of foci of swollen cells takes much longer.

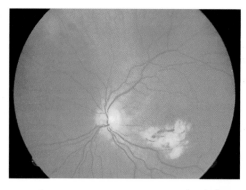

Fig. 11.6   Cytomegalovirus retinitis in an AIDS patient, showing triangular focus of retinal necrosis above the macula in the right fundus. (Photograph by Professor W R Lee, University of Glasgow.)

Serology: immunofluorescence or ELISA tests for IgM or IgG (to test for pre-existing immunity).

Treatment

(See also Chapter 18.)

Ganciclovir

Now widely used as a prophylactic or for treatment in immuno-suppressed patients, especially those with bone marrow transplants. Neutropenia is a fairly frequent complication of ganciclovir.

Foscarnet

Useful in the treatment of cytomegalovirus retinitis in AIDS patients.

EPSTEIN-BARR (EB) VIRUS

Epstein-Barr virus is named after the virologists who first observed it when examining cultures of lymphoblasts from Burkitt's lymphoma using the electron microscope. Infection is widespread in human populations, and most people have antibody to the virus by the time they reach adulthood.

Most infections are symptomless, especially if acquired during childhood: if infection is delayed until adult life there is greater likelihood of disease: this takes the form of *infectious mononucleosis* (glandular fever).

Persistence of virus: EB virus persists in latent form within lymphocytes following primary infection: the virus is present in cell cytoplasm in the form of unintegrated viral DNA. EB virus has oncogenic properties, and transforms cells in vitro.

Human cancer: EB virus has a strong association with Burkitt's lymphoma and nasopharyngeal carcinoma (see below).

Infectious mononucleosis

Clinical features

Incubation period: is long – 4–7 weeks.

Route of infection: close contact, mainly kissing: the virus is present in cells in salivary secretions. The disease is most prevalent among young adults, especially student populations (of whom a sizeable minority have no antibody).

Signs and symptoms: low-grade fever with generalized lymphadenopathy and sore throat due to exudative tonsillitis; malaise, anorexia and tiredness to a severe degree are characteristic; splenomegaly is common and most cases have abnormal liver function tests; a proportion have palpable enlargement of the liver and frank jaundice is not uncommon.

Mononucleosis: (or, more correctly, a relative and absolute lymphocytosis) is a diagnostic feature; at least 10% (and usually more) of the lymphocytes are atypical, with enlarged misshapen nuclei and excess cytoplasm; the atypical lymphocytes are both B and T cells, but mainly suppressor T cells stimulated in a cytotoxic response against EB virus-infected B cells.

Duration: in most cases of infectious mononucleosis, symptoms last 2–3 weeks but, in a proportion, tiredness and malaise persist for weeks or even months.

EB virus infection in the immunocompromised: can cause severe lymphoproliferative disease, which may be fatal and is characterized by infiltration of organs and tissues by immature B lymphocytes.

Purtillo's syndrome: fatal infectious mononucleosis, with malignant lymphoma due to EB virus, has been described in boys who suffer from this rare, congenital X-linked lymphoproliferative syndrome which is associated with immunodeficiency.

Diagnosis

Paul-Bunnell test: heterophil antibodies to sheep erythrocytes appear in the blood in infectious mononucleosis: this antibody can be absorbed by ox erythrocytes, but not by guinea-pig kidney. Haemagglutination with sheep erythrocytes and differential absorption with ox erythrocytes and guinea-pig kidney constitute the Paul-Bunnell test. Development of other nonspecific antibodies (e.g. rheumatoid factor and anti-i cold agglutinin) are also features of the disease.

EB virus antibody: is produced during infection but antibody is usually present before symptoms develop; the detection of IgM to virus capsid antigen and of antibody to early antigen are useful diagnostic tests.

Human cancer

Burkitt's lymphoma

A highly malignant tumour common in African children. Primarily a tumour of lymphoid tissue, but the earliest manifestations are often large tumours of the jaw and, in girls, sometimes of the ovaries; it spreads rapidly, with widespread metastases.

There is a striking geographical distribution: Burkitt's lymphoma is virtually confined to areas in Africa with holoendemic malaria and in which disease-carrying mosquito vectors are found. Outside Africa, e.g. in Western Europe and the USA, reported cases are sporadic and rare. The geographical distribution may be because malaria can act as a cofactor with EB virus, to produce malignant transformation in lymphoid tissue.

Nasopharyngeal carcinoma

This also shows a striking geographical and probably racial distribution, and is particularly common among the southern Chinese. Nasopharyngeal carcinoma is also associated with EB virus, and virus DNA is regularly present in the malignant epithelial cells of the tumour.

Virology

1. Double-stranded DNA virus
2. Grows in suspension cultures of human lymphoblasts.

Diagnosis

Serology:
Paul-Bunnell or *Monospot* test
Demonstration of EB virus-specific IgM by immunofluorescence test, with viral capsid antigen and antibody to early antigen.
Haematology: demonstration of atypical lymphocytes in the peripheral blood.

HUMAN HERPESVIRUS 6 (HHV 6)

Discovered in recent years, HHV 6 is a latent infection of lymphoid tissue. Infection is widespread, since there is a high incidence of antibody in normal populations, and it is acquired in early life.

Clinical features

Pathogenicity: still unclear: most infections appear to be symptomless.
Exanthema subitum (also known as *roseola infantum*): a mild facial rash in small babies is associated with HHV 6 infection.
Mononucleosis with cervical lymphadenopathy: has been described in a few adults undergoing primary infection.
Immunocompromised: can cause hepatitis in transplant patients, in whom viral reactivation has been reported – sometimes with fever and signs of generalized infection.

HUMAN HERPES VIRUS 7 (HHV 7)

Recently described, but so far without any disease association: infection is widespread (as judged by the prevalence of antibody) and acquired in childhood, although not as early in life as HHV 6 is acquired.

HUMAN HERPES VIRUS 8 (HHV 8)

This virus, recently discovered, is found (or at least traces of its DNA are found) in the cells of Kaposi's sarcoma in AIDS patients. Its role in the tumour is unclear – it may be causal, but this remains unproven.

12. Childhood fevers

Measles, mumps, and rubella are, with varicella, the common childhood fevers. Measles has been, at least partially, controlled by vaccination since 1968. Until 1988 in the UK, rubella vaccination was aimed at protecting girls in their teens against the risk of fetal infection while not interfering with naturally acquired immunity. In 1988, infant immunization with a combined, live, attenuated measles, mumps and rubella (MMR) vaccine was introduced. All these diseases are now in sharp decline in countries with national immunization programmes.

Erythema infectiosum is another childhood fever; due to human parvovirus B19.

MEASLES

Clinical features

Measles is now generally a mild disease in the UK, although complications used to be relatively frequent: in developing countries (especially in Africa) it is a severe disease and an important cause of childhood mortality and morbidity.

Incubation period: 10–14 days.

Prodromal symptoms are respiratory, e.g. nasal discharge and suffusion of the eyes.

The main illness is fever, with a maculopapular rash lasting 2–5 days (Fig. 2.1): the rash is an enanthema (as well as an exanthema) and characteristic spots (Koplik's spots) in the buccal mucosa inside the cheek and mouth are a diagnostic feature.

Immunity following natural infection is life-long: but note, measles itself has a suppressive effect on the immune system – especially on cell-mediated immunity.

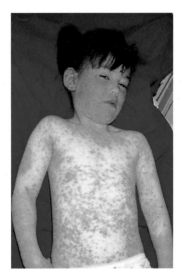

Fig. 12.1 Child with measles, showing characteristic rash: note the intensity of the dusky red maculopapular rash on the face. (Photograph by Dr A K Chaudhuri.)

Complications

Respiratory: the most common: bronchitis, bronchiolitis, croup and bronchopneumonia; may involve otitis media. Before the advent of antibiotics, these complications were largely responsible for the mortality associated with measles.

Giant cell pneumonia: a rare complication, seen in immuno-deficient children or those with chronic debilitating disease; due to direct invasion of the lungs by measles virus and usually fatal: there are numerous multinucleated giant cells in the lungs at post-mortem.

Neurological: two types of encephalitis are seen:

1. *Subacute sclerosing panencephalitis*: a rare, severe, chronic, neurological disease seen in children and young adults. Presents with personality and behavioural changes and intellectual impair-ment; progresses to convulsions, myoclonic movements, increasing neurological deterioration, leading to coma and death. Caused by persistent infection with defective measles virus following primary (and usually uncomplicated) measles several years previously; affected children have high titres of measles antibody in their serum and both IgM and IgG measles-specific antibody in the CSF. At post-mortem, there are numerous intranuclear inclusions

throughout the brain: measles virus can be grown from brain tissue.

2. *Post-infectious encephalitis*: follows measles in about one in every 1000 cases; the mortality rate can be as high as 50% and many survivors have residual neurological symptoms: commonly presents with drowsiness, vomiting, headache and convulsions. Virus is not demonstrable in the CNS.

Epidemiology

The attack rate in measles is high: before vaccination, virtually everybody in Britain under 15 years old had had the disease. When introduced into isolated communities, where the disease was not endemic and the entire population was susceptible, attack rates of more than 99% have been recorded.

Transmission is by inhalation of respiratory secretions from patients.

Epidemics: measles in Britain used to appear in epidemics every second year. Its prevalence has now declined sharply due to the introduction of measles vaccine, with a further marked reduction in cases since then, presumably due to the excellent uptake of MMR vaccine after it became part of the infant immunization programme in 1988.

Virology

1. Paramyxovirus, one serological type
2. RNA virus: single-strand negative-sense RNA
3. Enveloped particles, rather large – 120–250 nm; helical symmetry
4. Haemagglutinates and haemolyzes monkey erythrocytes
5. Grows in human embryo lung cells and primary monkey kidney cells, with syncytial CPE of multinucleated giant cells.

Diagnosis

Serology: complement fixation test; detection of measles IgM by immunofluorescence. In subacute sclerosing panencephalitis, by demonstration of measles antibody in the CSF.

Direct demonstration: of viral antigen by immunofluorescence in nasopharyngeal aspirates.

Isolation: rarely done.

Prophylaxis

Normal immunoglobulin contains measles antibody and can be used to confer immediate immunity to infants and to other unusually vulnerable individuals (e.g. the immunocompromised) who have been in contact with cases of measles.

MUMPS

Mumps is a generalized infection by a virus with a predilection for the CNS (*neurotropism*) and for glandular tissue.

Clinical features

Incubation period: relatively long: 14–21 days.

   Classical mumps is a febrile illness, with parotitis causing characteristic swelling of parotid and submaxillary glands (Fig. 12.2).

   Aseptic meningitis: mumps is an important cause of viral meningitis (and less often, meningoencephalitis), occasionally with muscular weakness or paralysis. Mumps meningitis is not

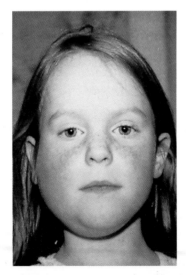

Fig. 12.2   Child with mumps, showing swelling of the parotid and submandibular glands on the right-hand side of the face. (Photograph by Dr A K Chaudhuri.)

accompanied by parotitis in 50% of cases. Nerve deafness is a rare complication.

Immunity: an attack is followed by solid and long-lasting immunity; second attacks are very rare.

Complications

Orchitis, pancreatitis and – rarely – oophoritis and thyroiditis are seen with mumps: about 20% of adult males who contract mumps develop orchitis.

Adults: tend to have more severe disease: orchitis and oophoritis are more common after puberty.

Epidemiology

Transmission: is by inhalation of infectious respiratory secretions.

Seasonal prevalence: most common in winter and spring.

Age distribution: more common in children from 5 to 15 years old, but not uncommon in young adults.

Infectiousness: less infectious than measles; as a result, infection in childhood is less common and a significant proportion of adults are non-immune.

Epidemics of mumps used to be seen every 3 years, followed by years when the prevalence of infection was low. MMR vaccine is having an impact and the incidence of mumps is now very low.

Virology

1. Paramyxovirus, one serological type
2. RNA virus: single-strand negative-sense RNA
3. Enveloped particles, rather large – 110–170 nm; helical symmetry
4. Haemagglutinates fowl erythrocytes
5. Grows in amniotic cavity of chick embryo and in monkey kidney and other tissue cultures, with haemadsorption.

Diagnosis

Serology: the most useful test: complement fixation test: two antigens are used: 'V' or viral surface protein: associated with long-lasting immunity; and 'S' or 'soluble' nucleoprotein: 'S' antibody appears early but fades early: useful for diagnosing acute infection.

Isolation: mainly used for diagnosis of mumps meningitis:
Specimens: CSF, possibly throat washings.
Inoculate: monkey kidney tissue cultures.
Observe: for haemadsorption of fowl erythrocytes.
Type virus: by inhibition of haemadsorption or haemagglutinin in tissue culture medium.

RUBELLA

Rubella is a mild disease, but if contracted in early pregnancy the virus can cause severe congenital abnormalities and disease in the fetus.

Clinical features

A mild febrile illness with a macular rash which spreads down from the face and behind the ears; there is usually pharyngitis and enlargement of the cervical – especially the posterior cervical – lymph glands. Infection is symptomless in some cases.

Incubation period: 14–23 days (average 18 days).

Virus is present in both blood and pharyngeal secretions, and is shed during the incubation period for up to 7 days before the appearance of the rash, and for 2 weeks after the rash appears.

Immunity after rubella: good, after both naturally- and vaccine-acquired rubella, but it is not solid and reinfections are well documented. Rarely, congenital infections have been reported as a result of maternal reinfection.

Complications

Rare: post-infectious encephalitis, thrombocytopenic purpura and arthralgia (painful joints).

Congenital infection

The teratogenic properties of the virus were first discovered in Australia in 1941, when Gregg (an ophthalmologist) noticed an increased number of cases of congenital cataract following an epidemic of rubella: affected infants had been born to mothers with a history of rubella in early pregnancy.

Congenital defects occur only if the mother has rubella in the first 16 weeks of pregnancy: after that rubella does not damage the fetus.

The main defects are a triad of:

- Cataract
- Nerve deafness
- Cardiac abnormalities (e.g. patent ductus arteriosus, ventricular septal defect, pulmonary artery stenosis, Fallot's tetralogy).

However, affected infants also have generalized infection which, together with the defects, is known as the *rubella syndrome* (Fig. 12.3). The signs of this are: hepatosplenomegaly, thrombocytopenic purpura, low birth weight, mental retardation, jaundice, anaemia and lesions in the metaphyses of the long bones.

The incidence of both deafness and defective vision increase as congenitally infected children grow up – doubtless due to easier recognition of these defects in older children.

The incidence of defects after maternal rubella in the first 3 months of pregnancy has varied from 10% to 54% in different

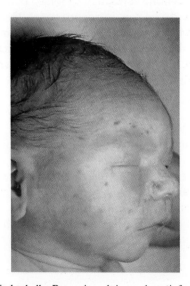

Fig. 12.3   Congenital rubella. Purpuric rash in newborn infant with congenitally-acquired rubella, who was subsequently found to have congenital heart disease and cataract as well. (Reproduced, with permission, from Topley and Wilson's Principles of Bacteriology, Virology and Immunity, 7th edn 1984. Edward Arnold, London, vol 4.)

studies. Maternal rubella at this time is also associated with a higher proportion of abortions and stillbirths.

Time of infection: the severity and multiplicity of defects are increased when infection is in the earliest weeks of pregnancy.

Immunity: infants with the rubella syndrome have IgM antibody to rubella virus and therefore are immunologically competent (the maternal antibody which crosses the placenta is IgG antibody).

Subacute sclerosing panencephalitis: has been reported as a rare, late, complication of congenital rubella.

Epidemiology

Age: mainly seen in children under 15 years old. Before the introduction of vaccination programmes, a proportion of people reached adult life without being infected and about 15% of women of child-bearing age were non-immune.

In the UK: following low-incidence years in 1991 and 1992, 1993 saw a resurgence, mostly in young adult males: males, of course, were only vaccinated from 1988, when the MMR vaccination programme became national policy. Rubella has shown a marked decline in incidence since the introduction of MMR vaccine – however, this is less striking than that observed with measles, perhaps because the previous policy of vaccinating girls has resulted in a relatively large cohort of unvaccinated and non-immune males born before 1988.

Virology

1. A non-arthropod-borne togavirus, one serological type
2. RNA virus: single-strand negative-sense RNA
3. Pleomorphic, enveloped particles, medium size – 50–75 nm; helical symmetry
4. Haemagglutinates avian erythrocytes
5. Grows in a rabbit kidney cell line (RK 13) with production of CPE, and in other tissue cultures, but without CPE.

Diagnosis

Mainly used to confirm suspected rubella in a pregnant woman or congenital rubella, and to detect non-immune pregnant women (tested when attending antenatal clinics).

Serology:

IgM antibody: recent infection is best diagnosed by detection of IgM by ELISA or immunofluorescence.

Single radial haemolysis: widely used for detecting immunity in pregnant women or in women at special risk, e.g. children's nurses, schoolteachers: it does not measure antibody titre and is less useful for the diagnosis of rubella.

Isolation: used for the diagnosis of congenital rubella in the fetus: now being replaced by PCR to detect rubella virus RNA or RNA fragments.

Inoculate: RK 13 (rabbit kidney) or SIRC (rabbit cornea) cell lines.

Observe: for CPE.

Prophylaxis

Passive immunization with normal immunoglobulin has possibly some attenuating effect or prophylactic effect in rubella: consider for use in maternal rubella if termination is unacceptable.

MMR VACCINATION

The MMR vaccination programme aims to eradicate measles, mumps and rubella from Britain. A high uptake of vaccine – which is being achieved – will increase herd immunity to the level at which too few susceptible hosts remain for the three viruses to survive in the community.

MMR vaccine

Indications: given to all children in the second year of life, with a booster at school-entry. In 1994 a nation-wide programme to immunize the whole school population was undertaken, to prevent an impending measles epidemic: in this it was successful.

Contains: live, attenuated measles, mumps and rubella virus strains.

Administration: one dose, subcutaneously or intramuscularly.

Protection: apparently excellent: immunity seems to be long-lasting, but careful surveillance will be necessary to monitor whether immunity persists over many years: there is evidence that immunity to measles after one dose of vaccine wanes, with cases appearing in adolescents.

Reactions: generally mild: fever, malaise, rash, coryza (due to the measles virus component); sometimes with parotitis and arthralgia (associated with the mumps and rubella virus components respectively); febrile convulsions.

Mumps meningoencephalitis: has been associated with one of the two vaccine strains used (the Urabe): vaccine used in the UK now contains the Jeryl Lynn strain.

Contraindications

- Pregnancy: must be avoided for 1 month after vaccination
- Immunodeficiency: due to immunosuppressive therapy, disease (leukaemia, other malignant disease) or other causes
- Hypersensitivity to eggs.

ERYTHEMA INFECTIOSUM (B19 INFECTION)

This disease (also called *slapped cheek* or *fifth disease*) is due to the human parvovirus B19.

Clinical features

Signs and symptoms: fever, erythematous rash, most intense on the cheeks where there is marked redness, hence the name 'slapped cheek disease', with circumoral pallor. The rash on the body and limbs becomes maculopapular: lesions fade from the centre leaving the periphery red, so developing a characteristic reticular or lace-like pattern. There is mild generalized lymphadenopathy and, especially in women, arthralgia with swelling and pain in the joints. Clinically, the disease resembles rubella.

Aplastic crises: B19 virus has a predilection for the haemopoietic cells of the bone marrow, causing aplastic crises: mainly described in children with chronic haemolytic anaemias such as sickle cell anaemia, hereditary spherocytosis, thalassaemia. There is evidence that previously healthy people also show transient bone marrow 'arrest' during the course of infection.

Symptomless infection: appears to be common – probably around 20% of those infected have no symptoms.

Non-immune hydrops fetalis: B19 virus can infect the fetus during the course of maternal infection. Many congenital infections are symptomless and the fetus develops normally – however, especially from the 10th to the 20th week of pregnancy, when the fetus seems most vulnerable, the virus can cause severe fetal infection and death, with a catastrophic fall in the haemoglobin level. The affected fetus resembles the hydrops fetalis associated with rhesus blood group incompatibility, so the parvovirus syndrome is called *non-immune* hydrops fetalis.

Immunodeficiency: persistent B19 infection, causing chronic anaemia, has been reported in children with leukaemia and other forms of immunodeficiency: also reported in patients with organ transplants.

Epidemiology

Epidemics: outbreaks of infection are seen in the community approximately every 4 years. Between outbreaks, B19 virus is endemic, causing sporadic infection.

Transmission: by inhalation of infected respiratory secretions.

Seasonal prevalence: most common in late winter and early spring.

Age: the peak incidence of infection is in childhood, during the early school years – from 5 to 10 years old.

Virology

1. Human parvovirus B19 is classed in the genus of autonomously replicating parvoviruses; other parvoviruses are defective and require helper viruses for replication.
2. DNA virus: single-stranded DNA. The virus genetic organization is interesting, because populations of virus show, in roughly equal measure, particles which contain either positive- or negative-sense DNA molecules.
3. Electron microscopy: small featureless icosahedral particles, 18–26 nm in diameter.
4. Haemagglutinates
5. Grows in tissue culture cells, but with difficulty, and needs specialized techniques.

Diagnosis

Serology: ELISA (or radioimmunoassay) for virus-specific IgM.

Direct demonstration: of viral DNA in tissues and blood, by PCR and DNA probe.

13. Poxvirus diseases

Most, possibly all, animal species are hosts to their own pox-viruses. The human poxvirus was smallpox – one of the most fatal of all virus infections: yet it was defeated, for three reasons:

1. Humans were the only hosts
2. There was an effective vaccine against it (originally discovered by Jenner (Fig. 13.1) in 1796)
3. By the mid-20th century there were only a limited number of areas of endemic infection.

Clinical features

Smallpox

Now eradicated: was a severe febrile illness characterized by a profuse vesicular rash and a high mortality (around 30%): survivors were left with disfiguring facial scars.

Eradication: in 1967 the World Health Organization embarked on a smallpox eradication campaign. This was based on a policy of 'search and containment', i.e. the isolation of cases and the tracing and vaccination of contacts. There was continuing and long-term surveillance of previously endemic areas before these were declared smallpox-free. The main endemic areas were India, Pakistan and Bangladesh and, in Africa, Ethiopia and Somalia. The campaign was outstandingly successful and smallpox has now been eradicated: the World Health Organization declared the world free of smallpox in May 1980. Destruction of the last re-maining stocks of virus (held in only two laboratories) is planned for the near future.

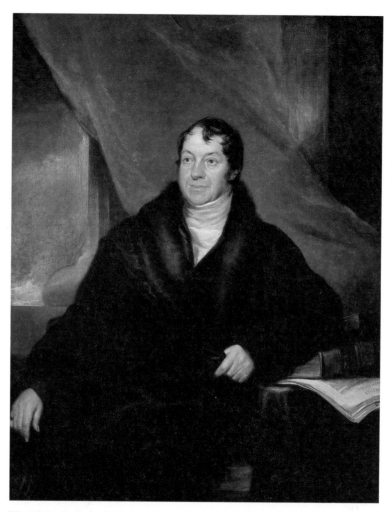

Fig. 13.1   Portrait of Edward Jenner, discoverer of the vaccination against smallpox. (Reproduced with the permission of the Royal Society of Medicine Press Ltd., London.)

Molluscum contagiosum

A low-grade infection in humans, characterized by reddish, waxy papules on the skin – usually in the axilla or on the trunk: a fairly common infection in children, spread by close contact, e.g. at swimming pools. Lesions contain numerous poxvirus particles, visible on electron microscopy; the lesions resolve spontaneously in 4–6 weeks: sometimes disseminates in immunocompromized patients (e.g. with AIDS).

Orf (contagious pustular dermatitis)

An infection of sheep and goats: occasionally transmitted to hands of animal workers, causing chronic granulomatous lesions: diagnosed by characteristic oval particles with criss-cross surface banding, seen on electron microscopy.

Paravaccinia (pseudocowpox)

The virus is similar to orf virus, but causes lesions on udders of cows and is occasionally transmitted to hands of animal workers.

Monkeypox

This is a disease resembling mild smallpox, which is due to a natural poxvirus of monkeys. It is seen in West Africa among people with frequent contact with monkeys – however, the main animal reservoir seems to be squirrels.

Tanapox

This virus is probably also acquired from contact with monkeys and, in humans, produces scanty vesicular lesions on the skin which do not progress to pustules. Outbreaks have been reported in East Africa.

Virology

1. Human poxviruses include smallpox (variola), alastrim (a milder form of smallpox, due to a related but distinguishable virus known as variola minor) and molluscum contagiosum. (Vaccinia virus, used for vaccination against smallpox, is of uncertain origin.)
2. DNA viruses: double-stranded DNA
3. Large viruses – approximately 250–300 nm: two morphological types of particle:
   - large, brick-shaped (vaccinia, molluscum contagiosum)
   - large, oval with criss-cross surface bonding (orf, paravaccinia)

4. Some grow in tissue cultures, others do not (e.g. molluscum contagiosum)
5. Many produce pocks on the chorioallantoic membrane of the chick embryo.

14. Viral hepatitis

Hepatitis is seen in many viral diseases – usually as part of a generalized infection: these include yellow fever, cytomegalovirus and Epstein-Barr infection, and congenital rubella. However, some viruses primarily target the liver to cause the disease *viral hepatitis*. The six hepatitis viruses are listed in Table 14.1.

Viral hepatitis presents a similar clinical picture even when due to different viruses. Sensitive and reliable laboratory tests, however, can now differentiate between them and this is important for prognosis.

General features of viral hepatitis

Symptoms: jaundice (Fig. 14.1) with low grade fever, anorexia,

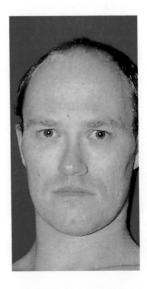

Fig. 14.1 Jaundice due to acute viral hepatitis: the sclera show typical yellow discoloration. (Photograph by Dr A K Chaudhuri.)

Table 14.1 Hepatitis viruses

Virus	A	B	C	D	E	G
Family	Picornavirus	Hepadnavirus	Flavivirus	Unclassified	?Calicivirus	Flavivirus
Genome	SS positive-sense RNA	DS DNA	SS positive-sense RNA	RNA (defective-hepatitis B acts as helper)	SS positive-sense RNA	SS positive-sense RNA
Transmission	faecal-oral, food, water, blood products	sexual; parenteral via blood, perinatal	parenteral via blood	as for hepatitis B	faecal-oral water-borne	parenteral via blood
Chronic hepatitis	No	Yes	Yes	Yes (increases risk of chronicity with hepatitis B)	No	No

SS: single-stranded; DS: double-stranded.
Hepatitis F virus may not exist.

nausea and malaise – the latter symptoms may precede the jaundice. Jaundice: obstructive in type with raised bilirubin, dark bile-containing urine and pale stools.

Transaminases: liver function tests are abnormal, with raised transaminase levels, e.g. ALT (alanine aminotransferase) in the serum.

Duration: variable, but usually 2–3 weeks.

Anicteric hepatitis: seen in all forms of viral hepatitis: with disturbance of liver function tests, fever, and the other constitutional signs and symptoms, but no frank jaundice.

Symptomless infection: is also common: a particular problem to control, because virus excretion may not be recognized.

Complications

1. **Fulminant hepatitis with massive liver necrosis** ('acute yellow atrophy'), leading to liver failure, coma and, very often, death. A rare complication of hepatitis A, somewhat more common with hepatitis B and a particular problem in pregnancy with hepatitis E.

2. **Chronic hepatitis**: may follow hepatitis B and hepatitis C (see below).

3. **Primary hepatocellular carcinoma**: chronic hepatitis B and C can lead to liver cancer.

HEPATITIS A

Clinical features

Incubation period: about 2–6 weeks.

Age incidence: mainly children 5–15 years old: but food-borne outbreaks often predominantly affect adults.

Clinically: milder than hepatitis B; fulminant hepatitis is a rare complication: overall case fatality rate in hepatitis A is 0.1%.

Alimentary infection: site of entry and primary multiplication is the gut: virus then spreads to infect the liver, where it multiplies in hepatocytes.

Excretion: virus is excreted in the faeces for about 2 weeks before the onset of jaundice, but for only up to 8 days after the onset of symptoms.

Viraemia: blood is briefly infectious, but is an uncommon source of infection.

Antibody: appears at the time of onset of jaundice.

Epidemiology

Distribution: world-wide: endemic in most countries and especially common in the tropics. Outbreaks appear from time to time, some of which are associated with faecal contamination of food or water.

Transmission: two main routes of infection:

1. *Case-to-case spread* via the faecal–oral route: the most common route of the spread of the disease; symptomless excretors are an important – because undetected – source of infection.

2. *Via contaminated food and water*: numerous outbreaks have been described, due to contamination of foodstuffs, by food-handlers excreting virus, or due to pollution of water by infected sewage. Raw shellfish (especially oysters), contaminated by growing in sewage-polluted water, have been responsible for several outbreaks.

Blood: recent outbreaks in haemophiliacs have been traced to contamination of batches of factor VIII – a reminder that hepatitis A involves a period of viraemia.

Seasonal prevalence: infection is more common in autumn and winter.

Decline: the incidence of hepatitis A increased during the late 1980s in the UK, to reach a peak in 1990, but has since declined sharply: the reasons for this are unclear. The decrease in incidence has not been observed in developing or tropical countries, where the prevalence is always higher than in developed countries.

Virology

1. A picornavirus
2. RNA: single-strand positive-sense RNA
3. Small spherical particles, 27 nm
4. Grows in tissue culture, but needs specialized techniques
5. Infects chimpanzees and certain other primates.

Diagnosis

Serology: detection of virus-specific IgM by ELISA.

Prophylaxis

Hepatitis A vaccine

A vaccine is now available for those at special risk, e.g. travellers and staff and patients of institutions for the mentally handicapped.

Contains: inactivated virus.

Administration: one dose injected intramuscularly, with optional booster 6–12 months later.

Protection: good: one dose gives immunity for a year, two doses give 10 years' protection.

Side-effects: mostly mild reactions at site of injection.

Passive immunization

Normal immunoglobulin protects people exposed to hepatitis A. There is no immunity for 2 weeks after inoculation, but the immunity thereafter lasts for 4 months: now being replaced by vaccination where possible.

HEPATITIS B

Clinical features

Incubation period: long – from 2 to 3 months, sometimes much longer.

Incidence: predominantly males.

Onset: typically rather insidious. good & Harmful way

Clinical course: generally a more severe disease than hepatitis A.

Viraemia: virus and virus surface antigen (see below) are present in the blood during the acute phase and can persist for longer.

Carriers: 5–10% of infected adults become long-term carriers, but the incidence of carriage in perinatally-infected babies is much higher: about 90%. In the UK, the prevalence of carriage is 0.1% but in Africa and Asia it is higher, ranging up to 20% in some areas.

Epidemiology

Hepatitis B used to be a major cause of post-transfusion hepatitis in Britain, but is now rare as a result of screening blood donations. Blood is highly infectious and minute traces can infect, e.g. by the use of communal or inadequately sterilized syringes and needles. Although rarely, infection has been transmitted from infected surgeons to patients during invasive surgery.

Drug abusers are at particular risk from hepatitis B. Infection is transmitted by sharing of syringes used for intravenous drugs: infection is endemic in the drug-abusing community.

Sexual transmission: an important route of infection, especially amongst male homosexuals.

Haemophiliacs: used to be at high risk because of contaminated factor VIII: no longer a problem due to screening of blood donations.

Renal dialysis units: in the past, hepatitis B was a particular problem in renal units: screening of blood donations, together with precautions to prevent cross contamination of equipment, have controlled this.

Tattooing and acupuncture: have also been the source of outbreaks.

Non-parenteral spread: some cases of hepatitis B, especially in young children, appear to be due to non-parenteral transmission – possibly through close personal contact.

Pregnancy: infection is readily passed from mother to infant, probably in the perinatal period rather than transplacentally in utero: the risk is increased if the mother has had acute hepatitis B during pregnancy and, if a carrier, is e antigen-positive (see below).

Sequelae

Persistent infection

Persistent infection is a common sequela of hepatitis B. It takes the form of:

1. *Symptomless carriage*: with minimal signs of liver damage: especially common in tropical countries as a result of vertical transmission from mother to child, but follows acute hepatitis B in adults in the UK in around 5–10% of cases.

2. *Chronic hepatitis*: this can take two forms:

   a. *Chronic persistent hepatitis* is a benign and self-limiting disease which can follow hepatitis B; there are mild inflammatory signs in the liver, but symptoms are minor or absent.

   b. *Chronic active hepatitis* follows hepatitis B in around 3% of cases. This is a serious disease, with liver dysfunction and a fluctuating course leading, in 15–20% of cases, to cirrhosis and so to progressive liver failure. Hepatitis B is not the only cause of chronic active hepatitis – in fact probably only around 10% of cases are due to previous hepatitis B.

Liver cancer

Primary hepatocellular carcinoma is much more common in carriers of hepatitis B virus than in antigen-negative people. The virus DNA integrates into liver cell chromosomes (a prerequisite for oncogenicity). Hepatocellular cancer is rare in Europe but common in Africa and Asia, and hepatitis B virus is now recognized as a major cause of cancer world-wide. The animal counterparts of human hepatitis B virus, which cause tumours in the host species, provide further evidence of the oncogenicity of this family of viruses.

Virology

1. Hepadnavirus.

2. DNA virus: double-stranded DNA but with single-stranded regions.

3. Electron microscopy: see Figure 14.2: the virions of hepatitis B virus are roughly spherical particles (42 nm in diameter), known as *Dane particles*: they contain a particle-associated DNA

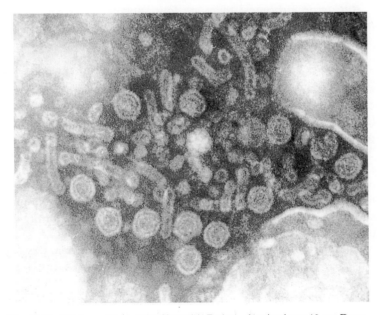

Fig. 14.2   Electron micrograph of hepatitis B virus, showing large 42 nm Dane particles, with smaller 22 nm spherical and tubular particles. × 220 000. (Photograph by Dr E A C Follett.)

polymerase; infected blood also shows 22 nm spherical particles – much more abundant than Dane particles – and tubular structures, both of which are aggregates of hepatitis B surface antigen (i.e. the virus coat protein).

4. Animals: diseases similar to human hepatitis B exist in the animal world, where species of ducks, squirrels and woodchucks are natural hosts to viruses which resemble hepatitis B in their properties. Liver cancer is associated with infection in woodchucks and ducks.

Antigenic structure

Hepatitis B virus has the following antigens:

1. **HBsAg**: (surface glycoprotein) antigen: found on the 22 nm particle and on the surface of the Dane particle
2. **HBcAg**: core antigen: the nucleoprotein core of the Dane particle
3. **HBeAg**: e antigen and part of the core protein of the Dane particle; associated with infectivity (see below).

Antigenic subtypes: there are four subtypes of HBsAg: *adw*, *adr*, *ayw* and *ayr*.

All share the group-specific determinant *a* in addition to allelic *d* and *y*, and *w* and *r* (which are mutually exclusive).

HBeAg is present – although briefly – in patients' blood in the acute phase of hepatitis B: presence in the blood of cases or carriers indicates active virus replication, and so correlates with infectivity of the blood. However, absence of e antigen does not mean that the blood concerned is non-infectious: in fact, around 20% of e antigen-negative carriers have circulating hepatitis B DNA and some, at least, are infectious. The continuing presence of e antigenaemia correlates with chronic liver disease and is found in the blood of a high proportion of patients with chronic active hepatitis following hepatitis B. Conversely, anti-e antibody in healthy carriers is evidence of low infectivity.

The three antigens and their antibodies are useful markers for the disease and its progression: summarized in Table 14.2.

Diagnosis

Serology: test by ELISA for HBsAg: if positive, test for anti-HBc IgM and for HBeAg: anti-HBc IgG without IgM is evidence of

Table 14.2 Markers of hepatitis B

	Acute infection	Convalescence	Carriers	Chronic hepatitis
HBsAg	+	–	+	+
HBeAg	+	–	+/–	+/–
Anti-HBc IgM	+	–	–	–
Anti-HBc IgG	+	+	+	+
Anti-HBs	–	+	–	–
Anti-HBe	–	+	+/–	+/–

past infection: anti-HBeAg indicates low infectivity. Anti-HBs IgG indicates immunity after vaccination.

Prophylaxis

Hepatitis B vaccine

Available for those at special risk, e.g. health care workers and close contacts (family or sexual) of cases or carriers, babies born to carrier or infected mothers, haemophiliacs, patients on renal dialysis, patients and staff in institutions for the mentally handicapped.

Contains: HBsAg, prepared by recombinant DNA technology: adsorbed onto aluminium hydroxide.

Administration: intramuscularly into the deltoid (not the gluteal muscle) in three doses: two, 1 month apart; the third, 6 months after the first.

Protection: good.

Response to vaccine: a significant proportion (10–20%) of vaccinees fail to respond. Vaccinees can be considered to be immune if antibodies are at least 100 mI units.

Safety: good.

Babies: born to HBsAg-positive mothers should be immunized within a few hours of birth: if the mother is HBeAg-positive, hepatitis B-specific immunoglobulin should be given simultaneously, but at a different site.

Passive immunization

Injection of hepatitis B-specific immunoglobulin gives partial but significant protection against the disease: can be used in people exposed in a single episode involving a high risk of infection, e.g.

accidental inoculation of blood suspected or known to contain hepatitis B virus: active immunization should be started as soon as possible.

Treatment

Chronic hepatitis B: interferon alfa reduces virus replication, and in around 10% of patients in one trial appeared to eliminate carriage: further studies are required to confirm the results long-term: the nucleoside analogues, lamivudine and famciclovir are also under trial.

HEPATITIS C

With effective control of transfusion-transmitted hepatitis B, it became apparent that not all transfusion hepatitis was due to hepatitis B. The main virus responsible for what was originally known as non-A-non-B hepatitis is now designated *hepatitis C*.

Clinical features

A milder disease than hepatitis B – only about 25% of patients have jaundice: generally with a shorter incubation period (usually 6–12 weeks).

    Antibody to the virus (at least that detected by current tests): develops relatively late – about 1–2 months (and sometimes longer) after exposure: antibody-positive patients are nearly always viraemic.

    Chronic hepatitis C: follows acute infection in about 60% of patients, of whom 20% go on to develop cirrhosis – but after an interval of around 10 years.

    Hepatocellular carcinoma: chronic hepatitis C is now recognized as an important cause of primary liver cancer, although this generally appears after a long time – around 20 years.

Epidemiology

Transmission: mainly transmitted parenterally by blood. Sexual transmission appears to be responsible for some cases in selected populations. Sporadic cases are also seen of which the route of infection is unknown.

    Blood donors: 0.1–0.5% in Britain have antibody to hepatitis C.

Haemophiliacs: many have evidence of past infection (i.e. presence of antiviral antibody), indicating contamination of factor VIII concentrate – now prevented by screening and treatment used in preparation of concentrates.

Pregnancy: around 10% of infected mothers transmit the virus to their babies.

Drug abusers: also have a high prevalence of antibody, indicating frequent exposure to infection through sharing of syringes.

Carriers: common: around half to three-quarters of cases of hepatitis C become long-term carriers of the virus in their blood.

Virology

The virus cannot be cultivated in cell culture, but it infects chimpanzees and virus-specific proteins have been genetically engineered from virus in infected chimpanzee blood: these form the basis of current tests for virus antibody. Features of hepatitis C virus:

1. Flavivirus: six genotypes are recognized
2. RNA genome: single-strand positive-sense RNA
3. Does not grow in cell culture
4. Infects chimpanzees.

Diagnosis

Serology: widely used for diagnosis in individual patients and also for screening blood donations: late seroconversion may mean cases are missed if tested only in the acute phase and in the immediate weeks following illness, by ELISA and using recombinant proteins (see above) and supplementary immunoblots (a version of the western blot technique).

Direct demonstration: PCR on blood samples detects viral RNA and indicates infectivity.

Treatment

Interferon alfa shows some benefit in cases of chronic hepatitis C: response is related to genotype, with cases of genotype 1b – common in Western Europe and the USA – being the poorest responders: requires further evaluation, as results of treatment are as yet disappointing.

HEPATITIS D (DELTA AGENT)

This interesting virus is defective, and can only replicate in the presence of a helper virus, hepatitis B, which supplies the necessary defective gene product. Hepatitis D is therefore found only in patients infected with hepatitis B.

Pathogenicity: unclear, but there is evidence that it increases the severity of hepatitis B.

Epidemiology

Hepatitis D virus is found among drug abusers infected with hepatitis B – and less often amongst other groups infected with hepatitis B. The ecology of the virus is unknown – for example, it is unclear how the virus maintains itself in populations, from where it originated, and so on. Some populations, e.g. in areas of South America, have a high prevalence of hepatitis D (and, of course, hepatitis B).

Virology

Little is known, apart from:

1. RNA genome: single-stranded RNA
2. Small particle coated with HBsAg and 35–37 nm in diameter.

Diagnosis

Serology: ELISA tests for antigen and antibody are available, but only in a few specialist laboratories.

HEPATITIS E

Hepatitis E is seen in community outbreaks (sometimes very large): transmission is faecal–oral, most often due to water-borne spread.

Clinical features

Incubation period: approximately 30–40 days.

Clinically: predominantly a disease of young adults, but of particular severity in pregnant women, in whom high case fatality rates have been recorded.

Geographical distribution: mainly seen in Asia, Africa and the Middle East. The extensive epidemic of water-borne hepatitis in Delhi in 1955 was probably due to hepatitis E. Rare in Britain.

Virology

1. RNA genome: single-stranded RNA
2. Particles morphologically similar to caliciviruses are seen in faeces of cases
3. Particles 27–34 nm in diameter
4. Transmissible to primates.

Diagnosis

Serology: due to recombinant DNA technology, an ELISA test for hepatitis E IgM and IgG antibody is available in a few centres, although not on a routine diagnostic basis.

HEPATITIS F AND G

Drug abusers and haemophiliacs: have a relatively high prevalence of antibody.

Role in disease: uncertain: may be non-pathogenic or may cause a few cases of post-transfusion hepatitis.

Hepatitis G virus is now identified, and at least partly characterized, by molecular technology: probably a flavivirus and similar to, although antigenically distinct from, hepatitis C; transmitted through blood transfusion.

Hepatitis F is a doubtful entity, and the virus may not exist at all.

15. Chronic neurological diseases due to viruses

Viruses cause chronic disease of the CNS (see Ch. 6): several are classified as '*slow virus diseases*', while others are chronic infections with conventional viruses. Slow virus diseases have a long incubation period, slow development of symptoms and a protracted, but eventually fatal, course. They are due to unconventional agents, which are now considered to be infectious proteins or *prions*.

Examples of chronic neurological diseases in humans due to conventional viruses are listed in Table 15.1. (Subacute sclerosing panencephalitis has been described in Chapter 12.) There are also many examples of chronic neurological disease in animals, due to a variety of different viruses.

PROGRESSIVE MULTIFOCAL LEUCOENCEPHALOPATHY

This rare disease is due to a papovavirus known as *JC*, one of two human polyomaviruses (the other is *BK virus*, and is not neurotropic). JC virus is 'opportunistic' in that it does not cause disease in normal people, but only causes disease in patients whose health is compromised by pre-existing disease, such as cancer or

Table 15.1 Chronic neurological virus diseases due to conventional viruses

Virus	Disease
Measles	Subacute sclerosing panencephalitis
Rubella	Subacute sclerosing panencephalitis (follows congenital infection)
JC (human polyomavirus)	Progessive multifocal leucoencephalopathy

leukaemia, or by immunosuppressive therapy. Progressive multi-focal leucoencephalopathy is a reactivation of JC virus latent in the brain.

BK virus is also an opportunistic pathogen, and has been isolated from immunodeficient patients, mainly from urine – sometimes in association with ureteric stenosis: due to reactivation of latent virus.

Clinical features

Varied neurological signs: such as hemiparesis, dementia, dysphasia, incoordination, impaired vision and hemianaesthesia.

Duration: usually fatal in 3–4 months.

Pathology: multiple foci of demyelination in cerebral hemi-spheres and cerebellum: brain stem and basal ganglia are also sometimes affected: oligodendrocytes with swollen nuclei and intranuclear inclusions are characteristic features.

Symptomless viruria: with either JC or BK virus, is not un-common in pregnancy – around 3–7% of pregnant women excrete human polyomaviruses; transplant patients also excrete these viruses, which apparently usually cause no urinary symptoms.

Epidemiology

Infection is common in the community since around 50–60% of adults in Britain have antibody to it. BK virus antibody is also present in a large proportion of human populations, so symptom-less infection seems to be widespread.

Virology

1. Papovavirus, in the genus polyomavirus
2. Genome is circular, double-stranded DNA
3. Electron microscopy: small icosahedral particles with 72 capsomeres; size 42–45 nm
4. Grows in human fetal glial tissue cultures
5. Haemagglutinates human and guinea-pig erythrocytes at 4°C.

SPONGIFORM ENCEPHALOPATHIES

These are neurological diseases due to unconventional agents and characterized by spongiform or vacuolating degeneration in the brain. All are transmissible to experimental animals, but their causal agents are clearly not typical viruses and have never been seen by electron microscopy: the current theory is that these agents are infectious proteins – *prions*.

The diseases show the following features:

1. Long incubation period
2. Protracted, severe, progressive course: always fatal
3. Pathology: degeneration of the CNS with status spongiosus
4. Lesions show no inflammatory reaction
5. No antibody or other immune response.

Four diseases of this type are listed in Table 15.2.

Prions

The spongiform encephalopathies are associated with the presence in the brain (and sometimes other tissues) of characteristic fibrils composed of a cell protein coded by a gene, the PrP gene, on the host cell chromosome. This protein (originally protease-resistant protein, now more often taken to mean prion protein) exists in abnormal form in the spongiform encephalopathies. Although still controversial, it seems that prions may represent a form of infectious protein: abnormal prions may combine with the normal cellular protein to induce replication of the abnormal form.

Prions are extremely resistant to heat and other inactivating agents.

Susceptibility: enhanced susceptibility to infection is associated with mutations in the PrP gene.

Table 15.2   Chronic neurological diseases due to unconventional agents

Disease	Host	Pathology	Disease syndrome
Creutzfeldt-Jakob	Human	Subacute degeneration of brain and spinal cord; status spongiosus of cortex	Presenile dementia; ataxia, spasticity, involuntary movements
Kuru	Human	Subacute cerebellar degeneration; status spongiosus	Postural instability; ataxia, tremor
Scrapie	Sheep	Subacute cerebellar degeneration	Ataxia, tremor, constant rubbing
Bovine spongiform encephalopathy	Cattle	Status spongiosus of brain	Ataxia, rubbing, fasciculation of muscles

CREUTZFELDT-JAKOB DISEASE (CJD)

A rare progressive neurological disease, characterized by a combination of presenile dementia and symptoms due to lesions in the spinal cord.

Clinical features

1. **Prodromal stage**: the disease starts with tiredness, apathy and vague neurological symptoms.

2. **Second stage**: the patient develops ataxia, dysarthria and progressive spasticity of the limbs; this is associated with dementia, and often involuntary movements such as myoclonic jerks or choreo-athetoid movements.

3. **Steady progression until death**: usually from about 6 months to 2 years after the onset of symptoms.

Pathology: diffuse atrophy with status spongiosus in the cerebral cortex; atrophy also in basal ganglia, cerebellum, substantia nigra and anterior horn cells.

New variant CJD: during 1996, a new type of CJD, *vCJD*, was reported: this affected a younger age group and was characterized by large kuru-like plaques in the brain: it was feared that this form of the disease might be due to the prion of bovine spongiform encephalopathy (BSE), ingested in beef and having crossed the species barrier from cow to humans. The variant appeared in 1994 and, by 1996, 14 cases had been reported.

Gerstmann-Straussler-Scheinker disease: an atypical form of CJD, most often seen as an inherited disorder, in which cerebellar ataxia is a feature: occasionally sporadic: also transmissible to primates.

Fatal familial insomnia is another human spongiform encephalopathy, of which little is presently known.

Causal agent

Transmission experiments: the disease is reproduced in chimpanzees and other primates after intracerebral inoculation of brain tissue from cases of the disease: the incubation period is 11–14 months; the disease can also be transmitted peripherally (by combined intravenous, intraperitoneal and intramuscular routes).

Human infection: the natural route of infection is unknown, but CJD has been accidentally transmitted from undiagnosed patients with the disease via corneal graft and by electrodes used for electroencephalography. Growth hormone derived from human pituitary gland has been responsible for many cases. Grafts of dura mater from cadavers have also transmitted the disease.

KURU

Kuru is a fatal human disease found only among the Foré-speaking people in New Guinea. It seems to have appeared about 60 years ago. The incidence increased up to the late 1950s, when kuru was responsible for about half the deaths of the Foré-speaking people. The incidence of kuru declined rapidly from the early 1960s, and it is now rare.

Clinical features

Kuru is a native word meaning 'trembling with cold and fever'.
Incubation period: around 4–20 years.
The disease has three stages:

1. The *first or ambulant* stage of the disease starts with unsteadiness in walking, postural instability, cerebellar ataxia and tremor; facial expressions are poorly controlled and speech becomes slurred and tremulous.

2. The *second or sedentary* stage is reached when the patient cannot walk without support, but can still sit upright unaided.

3. In the *tertiary stage* the patient cannot sit upright without clutching a stick for support: even a gentle push makes the patient lurch violently; the patient becomes progressively more paralysed and emaciated until death, which is due to bulbar depression or intercurrent infection.

Duration averages 1 year, but ranges from 3 months to 2 years.
Pathology: neuronal degeneration in cerebellum with astrocytic hyperplasia, gliosus and status spongiosus; demyelination is minimal or absent; amyloid plaques and fibrils are characteristic features.

Epidemiology

Incidence: kuru is uncommon in adult males; most patients are women or children of either sex.
Transmission: cannibalism of dead relatives is thought to have been responsible for the spread of kuru among the Foré

people. The women and children (but not men) eat the viscera and brains of relatives, including those who have died of kuru. Spread may have been through contact of infected tissues with abrasions on skin as well as ingestion. The tissues are inadequately cooked, so the causal agent would not be inactivated by cooking. Cannibalism stopped around 1957 and kuru has now declined sharply in incidence.

Transmission experiments: intracerebral inoculation of brain tissue from kuru victims into chimpanzees and other primates causes the animals to develop the symptoms of kuru after an incubation period of 2 years.

SCRAPIE

Scrapie is a neurological disease of British sheep, known to exist 200 years ago. Long recognized as infectious, it can be transmitted experimentally, not only to sheep but to laboratory mice and hamsters.

Clinical features

Natural scrapie affects both sheep and goats. The following are features of natural scrapie in sheep.

Long incubation period: 2–5 years.

Signs and symptoms: affected sheep suffer from excitability, incoordination, ataxia, tremor and continuous scratching or rubbing due to sensory neurological disturbance (Fig. 15.1); the symptoms progress to paralysis and death.

Pathology: cerebellar neuronal degeneration, with astrocytic proliferation and status spongiosus.

Heredity: a major gene controls whether or not sheep develop disease after experimental inoculation. The operation of the gene is complex: however, different strains of scrapie have distinctive incubation periods, indicating genetically-determined control over some features of the disease.

Route of infection: the disease seems to be maintained in flocks by vertical transmission from ewes to lambs, possibly mainly perinatally through contact with infected placentas.

TRANSMISSIBLE MINK ENCEPHALOPATHY

A disease also spread from sheep products and due to scrapie

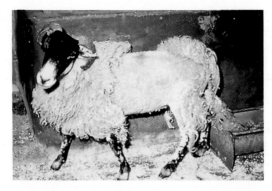

Fig. 15.1   Scrapie-infected sheep: the loss of fleece is due to rubbing ('scrapie') – a neurological rather than a dermatological disorder. (Photograph by M Stack, Pathology Research Discipline, Central Veterinary Laboratory, Weybridge.)

agent: mink bred in mink farms become infected when fed on the heads of scrapie-infected sheep.

BOVINE SPONGIFORM ENCEPHALOPATHY (BSE)

First recognized in 1986, and now a major epidemic disease in British cattle: thought to be due to scrapie transmitted from inadequately treated sheep carcasses, rendered down and used to supplement cattle feed as a source of protein.

Clinical features

Incubation period: 2.5–8 years.

Signs and symptoms: abnormal gait, ataxia, apprehension and anxiety, slipping and falling, licking nose: progresses to frenzy and aggression.

Duration: between 2 weeks and 6 months.

Pathology: degeneration with vacuolation, especially in medulla oblongata: neuronal loss and gliosis.

Epidemiology

Transmission to other animal species: BSE has been reported in some zoo animals – presumably the transmission is via scrapie-infected sheep offal in their feed: BSE has also appeared in domestic cats.

Epidemic: the disease in cattle is now declining sharply, but has not disappeared: although probably rare, transmission from infected cows to calves has been reported.

vCJD: the variant form of CJD may demonstrate transmission from infected beef across the species barrier to humans, but this is not yet proven.

16. Warts

Warts are one of the commonest virus infections, and few people reach adult life without suffering from them. Due to papillomaviruses, knowledge of their virology has come from modern biotechnology, since they cannot be cultivated in vitro.

Clinical features

Warts are benign tumours of the skin, with virus-induced proliferation of keratinized and non-keratinized squamous epithelium – i.e. both skin and mucous membranes.

Common warts: most common on hands and feet (plantar warts), they also infect the genitalia and anus, where they may be large and are known as *condylomata acuminata*; small, clinically symptomless warts are common in the female population; warts are also found in the larynx and oral cavity.

Table 16.1 lists the principal clinical types of wart and the papillomaviruses found in them.

Condylomata acuminata: a sexually-transmitted disease, in which the warts are occasionally very large (Fig. 16.1): rarely, and only in the immunocompromised, they become malignant, with change to invasive squamous epitheliomata.

Laryngeal papilloma: rare in Britain, but relatively common in other countries, e.g. southern USA: the juvenile form is acquired during birth from maternal condylomata acuminata: there is a tendency to recur after treatment.

Epidermodysplasia verruciformis: a rare autosomal recessive inherited disease, in which affected patients develop multiple warts with a high risk (around one-third) of malignant change to squamous cell carcinomata. Interestingly, the papillomaviruses responsible belong to several different and unusual types of virus: types 5 and 8 are the commonest found in the lesions.

149

Table 16.1   Human warts and the main papillomaviruses with which they are associated

Wart	Papillomavirus type
Plantar	1, 4
Hand	2
Flat; juvenile	3, 10
Condylomata acuminata	6, 11
Carcinoma of cervix	16, 18, 31
Laryngeal	6, 11
Warts and macules in epidermodysplasia verruciformis	5, 8 (and other types not found in other warts)
Butcher's warts	7

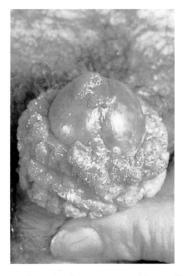

Fig. 16.1   Genital warts: large penile warts, caused by papillomavirus. (Photograph by The Photography and Illustration Centre, The Middlesex Hospital.)

Butcher's warts: an occupational hazard of slaughtermen and butchers: due to type 7 virus, which is not found in human populations and for which, to date, no animal source has been detected.

Epidemiology

Transmission: by contact, e.g. hand to hand; via water in the surrounds of swimming pools in the case of plantar warts on the feet; sexual transmission in the case of genital warts and via the infected mother's birth canal in the case of juvenile laryngeal papilloma.

Papillomaviruses and cancer

Papillomaviruses are now recognized as a cause – possibly in part acting with a cofactor – of cervical cancer (see below). Amongst animals (many, perhaps all, species of which have their own host-specific papillomaviruses), some papillomaviruses certainly cause cancer. In American cotton tail rabbits, the Shope papilloma, which is virus-induced, becomes cancerous in 25% of animals: in domestic rabbits, similar experimentally-induced Shope papillomata undergo malignant change at a much higher rate. Amongst cattle, alimentary papillomata – due to bovine papillomavirus type 4 – become malignant when the animals are fed on bracken, acting as a cofactor.

Human cancer

There is good evidence that papillomaviruses can cause human cancer: the viruses with greatest oncogenic potential are types 16 and 18, in cervical cancer.

Cervical cancer shows strong risk factors, such as early age at first intercourse, multiple sexual partners, high parity, etc.: the incidence of the disease correlates with high sexual activity (it is virtually unknown in nuns), and it therefore has some of the characteristics of a sexually-transmitted disease. Precancerous lesions, known as *cervical intraepithelial neoplasia (CIN)*, are seen in three degrees of histological change to malignancy. Lesions with the highest risk of developing into invasive cancer are CIN III, which contain DNA of types 16 and 18.

Skin cancer: apart from the warts associated with epidermodysplasia verruciformis, skin warts virtually never become malignant in immunocompetent people. Interestingly, warts are common in patients with renal transplants (who are, of course, immunocompromised) and in such patients the development of squamous cell cancer – associated with types 5 and 8 papillomaviruses – has been described.

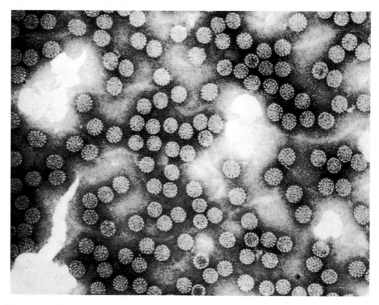

Fig. 16.2   Human papillomavirus. The virus particles have cubic symmetry.
× 90 000. (Photograph by Dr E A C Follett.)

Virology

1. Papovavirus family: papillomavirus genus: more than 60 types
   have been identified on the basis of DNA homology
2. DNA virus: with double-stranded, circular DNA
3. Electron microscopy: icosahedral particle with 72 capsomeres,
   52–55 nm in diameter (Fig. 16.2)
4. Host-specific: do not grow in any cell cultures: human
   papillomaviruses are not pathogenic for any animals.

Diagnosis

Laboratory diagnosis is not available for individual patients. The
viruses cannot be cultivated in vitro and have been studied by
molecular studies on the DNA in the warts themselves.

Typing: Papillomaviruses are typed by estimation of the degree
of DNA homology, by hybridization of their DNA with that of
other human papillomaviruses.

17. Retroviruses

The discovery of human retroviruses has been one of the most important developments in clinical virology. Retroviruses have long been known as the cause of cancer in various animal species: research into them has led to the discovery of the cause of AIDS – and to major advances in knowledge of the molecular basis of cancer.

ANIMAL RETROVIRUSES

Many retroviruses cause natural cancer in their animal host. They also produce leukaemia or sarcomata on inoculation into experimental animals. Although sarcoma viruses transform cells, most of the leukaemia viruses do not.

Morphology

Retrovirus particles show slight differences on electron microscopy:

1. *C-type particles*: most retroviruses have spherical enveloped particles, surrounded by spikes or knobs and containing a rounded central core composed of RNA and protein (Fig. 17.1).

2. *B-type particles*: mouse mammary tumour virus has particles similar to C-type particles, but with an eccentric core or nucleoid.

3. *D-type particles*: have typical retrovirus morphology but with a central wedge-shaped core, and are typified by HIV – the virus of human acquired immune deficiency syndrome (AIDS).

Note: all retrovirus particles contain the enzyme reverse transcriptase (see Ch. 2).

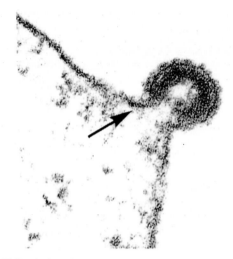

Fig. 17.1   Feline leukaemia virus: a typical C-type retrovirus particle, budding through the plasma membrane on its release from the cell. The continuity between the cell surface membrane and the virion is indicated by the arrow, and the spikes on the surface of the outer virion membrane are clearly seen. × 190 000. (Photograph by Dr Helen Laird.)

Genome structure

The retrovirus genome has three main genes:

1. The *gag* gene: codes for the core protein antigens of the virus particle. These are cleaved from a larger precursor protein.
2. The *pol* gene: codes for the protein that is the reverse transcriptase.
3. The *env* gene: codes for the envelope glycoproteins of the virion.

Long terminal repeat regions at each end of the genome contain powerful promoter and enhancer sequences: responsible for the integration of provirus – the DNA transcript of the viral genome RNA, produced by reverse transcriptase – into the cellular chromosome. Additional regulatory genes: *tat* (transactivating transcription), *rev*, *nef*, etc., are present in HIV.

Oncogenes

Many retrovirus genomes have *oncogenes* incorporated into their structure. Oncogenes are genes whose expression can be associated with tumour production, and which are present in many normal cells as a result of vertical inheritance.

Retroviruses cause cancer when their genome acquires cellular oncogenes by recombination. This happens when RNA tumour viruses integrate in the form of provirus DNA into cellular chromosomes. Numerous oncogenes have been described in animal retroviruses. In these cases their designation is preceded by the letter 'v', e.g. v-*myc* or v-*ras*: their cellular counterparts are known as c-*myc* or c-*ras*.

Oncogenes do not always give rise to carcinogenesis. They need to be activated, and different mechanisms can be responsible for this:

1. A **virus promoter**, such as that contained in the long terminal repeat regions of the retrovirus genome.

2. A **cellular promoter**: possibly by translocation of the oncogene to a site on a chromosome with high activity.

3. A **cofactor**, such as a chemical carcinogen.

4. **Interaction with other oncogenes**.

It seems likely that oncogenes normally function as regulatory mechanisms in cells: their activation to produce tumours is probably the result of a loss of control of normal gene function, leading to disturbance of the usual regulatory activity.

Epidemiology

Most animal species (including humans) in which a detailed search has been made are natural hosts for retroviruses. These are specific to the species concerned (Table 17.1).

Table 17.1   Animal tumour-producing retroviruses

Host	Virus	Tumour
Chicken	Rous sarcoma virus	Sarcoma
	Avian leukosis viruses	Fowl leukaemia
Mouse	Murine sarcoma virus	Sarcoma
	Murine leukaemia viruses	Leukaemia
	Mouse mammary tumour virus	·Breast cancer
Cat	Feline sarcoma virus	Sarcoma
	Feline leukaemia virus	Leukaemia
Cattle	Bovine leukaemia virus	Leukaemia
Primates	Simian sarcoma virus	Marmoset sarcoma
	Gibbon ape leukaemia virus	Gibbon ape leukaemia

Transmission from animal to animal takes place in three ways:

1. *Horizontal*: in which the virus spreads by close contact, or possibly inhalation, between infected and susceptible animals. This is an important route in naturally occurring infection in outbred animals not reared in a laboratory, such as cats.

2. *Vertical*: in which the virus spreads from mother to offspring either in utero, at birth, or via the mother's milk.

3. *Genetic*: a form of vertical transmission in which the virus is inherited as a provirus (or viral DNA transcript) integrated into the chromosomes of the germ cells of the parent animals. The viruses produced from these proviruses are known as *endogenous* viruses, and are typical retroviruses: some are tumour-producing on inoculation into experimental animals, but many are not. Endogenous retrovirus genes are usually repressed, but can be induced or derepressed by various agents, with production of virus in the animal. Endogenous retroviruses have been demonstrated in normal cells of chickens, mice, cats and primates. Retrovirus sequences have been identified in human chromosomes.

Tumours produced by retroviruses

Most retroviruses which cause tumours in animals are one of:

1. Sarcoma viruses
2. Leukaemia viruses.

Sarcoma viruses

Sarcoma viruses readily transform cells in tissue culture, and produce solid tumours – fibrosarcomata – on inoculation into animals of the host species. Most are defective, and in order to replicate require the presence of a helper virus (usually a leukaemia virus of the same animal species) to supply the product of the defective gene. The deletion often involves the *env* gene and, as a result, sarcoma viruses are antigenically similar to the helper leukaemia virus.

Leukaemia viruses

Leukaemia viruses produce leukaemia on inoculation into animals. Most do not transform cells in tissue culture, although some do so. Leukaemia viruses are not defective and generally replicate in tissue culture without CPE: cell growth and division are not affected. Table 17.1 lists some typical tumour-producing animal retroviruses, their host animal species and the tumours produced.

HUMAN RETROVIRUSES

Four human retroviruses have been discovered – see Table 17.2. All are tropic for CD4 helper T lymphocytes, but whereas HTLV-I and II transform and cause the T cells to proliferate, HIV-1 and 2 are cytopathic and kill the cells. The CD4 receptors on the T cells are the receptors for these viruses.

HTLV-I

HTLV-I is an endemic infection usually latent in T lymphocytes but, rarely, causing adult T cell leukaemia/lymphoma (leukaemias/lymphomas are mostly tumours of B lymphocytes). HTLV-I is also the cause of tropical spastic paraparesis.

Clinical features

Incubation period: symptoms appear after a prolonged period – usually many years.

T cell leukaemia/lymphoma: an aggressive malignancy of T cells, with lymphadenopathy and hepatosplenomegaly; sometimes cerebral involvement. The disease may present with lymphomatous infiltration of the skin (so that it can be mistaken clinically for mycosis fungoides). There is an increased level of calcium in the blood, which may be related to osteoporotic lesions in bones – another characteristic feature.

Table 17.2   Human retroviruses

Virus	Disease
Human T cell lymphotropic viruses	
HTLV-I	Adult T cell leukaemia/lymphoma; tropical spastic paraparesis
HTLV-II	Unknown
Human immunodeficiency virus	
HIV-1	AIDS (acquired immune deficiency syndrome)
HIV-2	AIDS

Tropical spastic paraparesis: a progressive, non-demyelinating spastic paralysis, more common in females than males.

Symptomless infection: most infected people do not develop disease, and the risk factors that lead to the onset of disease are unknown.

Virus is present as a latent infection in the T cells of infected individuals: atypical transformed T cells are present, sometimes in large numbers, in the peripheral blood of patients with T cell leukaemia/lymphoma.

Antibody persists throughout the infection.

Epidemiology

Geographical distribution: marked; infection is particularly common in south-western Japan, the Caribbean and West Africa. It is also present in Britain, mostly in immigrants from the West Indies.

Transmission: sexual, vertical (via infected breast milk) and by blood – transfused blood is highly infectious.

Seroprevalence: antibody to HTLV-I in endemic areas varies in prevalence, generally being around 1–5%, although clusters are found in which the prevalence is much higher. The prevalence of antibody in children is low, but rises with increasing age.

Virology

1. RNA virus with typical retrovirus genome structure
2. Electron microscopy: C-type particles
3. Grows in culture in human T lymphocytes stimulated with interleukin 2: cells are transformed or immortalized without cytopathic effect.

Diagnosis

Serology: ELISA, particle agglutination test, western blot – available at specialized laboratories.

HTLV-II

Originally isolated from a patient with hairy-cell leukaemia, the virus is now thought to be unrelated to this disease. Similar structurally and with extensive nucleic acid homology to HTLV-I, its epidemiology and pathogenicity are ill-understood. Clusters of antibody-positive people have been described amongst drug abusers in London, UK and in several cities in the USA, and also in certain other areas of the world, e.g. Africa, where infection seems endemic and unrelated to drug abuse.

HTLV-I and II can be distinguished serologically and by differences in their gene sequences using products of PCR.

HIV

HIV – the cause of AIDS – is at present the most intensively investigated virus. AIDS results from failure of the immune system, probably due to the cytopathic effect of HIV on T4 helper lymphocytes. Note that some animal retroviruses, for example, some variants of feline leukaemia virus, also cause immunodeficiency, so that AIDS-like disease is not unique to humans.

Human AIDS appears to be a genuinely new disease. The first infection recorded was in Kinshasa, Zaire, in 1959 (antibody to HIV was later detected in serum taken at that time). Since then, AIDS has become epidemic in Africa and, with a somewhat different epidemiology, in the USA and Western Europe. It has now been found in virtually every country in the world.

There are two types of virus: HIV-1, the main cause of the world-wide AIDS pandemic, and HIV-2, recently discovered in West Africa and, as yet, not showing significant spread from there.

Clinical features

The natural history of HIV has three stages:

1. *Acute primary infection*: often symptomless, but sometimes with an infectious mononucleosis-like illness some 2 weeks to 3 months after exposure with fever, rash, sore throat, night sweats, malaise, lymphadenopathy, diarrhoea, and relative and absolute lymphocytosis in the peripheral blood. There may be mouth and genital ulcers, and neurological symptoms are not uncommon. The symptoms subside spontaneously, and antibody appears at about this time.

2. *A variable symptomless period*: usually around 1–10 years, during which patients may show depressed counts of CD4 lymphocytes.

3. *Symptomatic stage*, leading into full-blown AIDS: often presents with persistent lymphadenopathy and constitutional upsets, together with a variety of infections and other conditions associated with defective cell-mediated immunity:

- Fever
- Diarrhoea
- Fatigue
- Candidiasis – oropharyngeal, vulvo-vaginal; persistent or frequent
- Zoster: two episodes, or one involving more than one dermatome
- Hairy leukoplakia of the tongue
- Idiopathic thrombocytopenic purpura.

Other conditions sometimes seen include: cervical dysplasia or CIN, listeriosis, pelvic inflammatory disease, peripheral neuropathy and bacillary angiomatosis (a rare infection of skin capillaries).

Progression to AIDS: correlates with decrease in CD4 lymphocyte count and the appearance of the internal core antigen, P24, in the blood.

AIDS

Characterized by an extreme degree of immunodeficiency, with low and decreasing CD4 counts. This results in a series of opportunistic infections, as microorganisms are uncontrolled by the patient's immune mechanisms and proliferate to cause a variety of unusually severe and persistent infections; certain tumours – Kaposi's sarcoma is particularly characteristic (Fig. 17.2) – are also features of AIDS. Indicator diseases for AIDS are shown in Table 17.3.

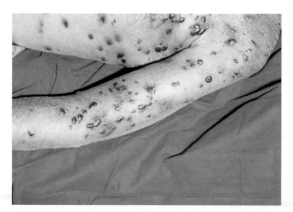

Fig. 17.2   AIDS. The characteristic purplish skin tumours of Kaposi's sarcoma. (Photograph by The Photography and Illustration Centre, The Middlesex Hospital.)

Table 17.3 AIDS: indicator infections

Infection	Disease
Parasites	
Pneumocystis carinii[a]	Pneumonia
Cryptosporidium	Diarrhoea
Isospora belli	Diarrhoea
Toxoplasmosis of brain	Encephalitis
Viruses	
Herpes simplex	Oral ulceration (prolonged); pneumonitis; oesophagitis
Cytomegalovirus	Pneumonia; retinitis
JC virus	Progressive multifocal leucoencephalopathy
Bacteria	
Mycobacterium avium complex	Extrapulmonary, disseminated disease
Mycobacterium tuberculosis	Tuberculosis: pulmonary, extrapulmonary
Salmonella spp	Septicaemia, recurrent
Fungi	
Candida albicans	Oesophageal, pulmonary
Coccidiomycosis	Extrapulmonary
Cryptococcus neoformans	Meningitis
Histoplasmosis	Disseminated
Tumours	
	Cervical cancer – invasive
	Kaposi's sarcoma
	Lymphoma; cerebral B-cell lymphoma
Other	
HIV	Encephalopathy/dementia
	Wasting disease
	Pneumonia, recurrent

[a]Recent molecular data suggest this may be a fungus rather than a parasite.

The disease is uniformly fatal, although treatment of HIV (by zidovudine (AZT) or other drugs) and treatment of the associated infections prolongs life.

Paediatric AIDS

Infected mothers: transmit HIV to their babies in approximately 20% of cases: the virus may spread to the child:

1. *Transplacentally* – to cause infection in utero
2. *During delivery* or in the perinatal period
3. *Through breastfeeding.*

Clinically, infected infants show the following signs and symptoms:

- Failure to thrive
- Fever
- Diarrhoea
- Frequent infections, including opportunistic and disseminated infections
- Lymphadenopathy
- Lymphoid interstitial pneumonia
- Parotitis
- Hepatosplenomegaly
- Neurological disease: most often a progressive encephalopathy, sometimes dementia, convulsions, motor disorders.

Although broadly similar to adult AIDS, lymphoid interstitial pneumonia and parotid gland enlargement are not seen in the adult disease.

Pathology

AIDS is often described as a disease of CD4 helper T lymphocytes, but although lymphoid tissues are clearly major targets for the virus (which attaches specifically to the CD4 receptors on lymphocytes and on cells such as macrophages), the virus causes disseminated infection and affects many organs, e.g. brain, gut, bone marrow and skin. The pathological processes involved in the course of the infection are still unclear.

Epidemiology

Transmission:

- Sexual
- Parenterally by infected blood or blood products, or by needle-sharing among drug abusers
- In utero from mother to child, perinatally or via breast milk.

Sources of virus: virus is present in blood, semen, vaginal secretions and breast milk.

High risk: given the routes of infection, certain categories of people are at high risk of infection:

- Promiscuous, i.e. those who often change sexual partners – especially male homosexuals
- Injecting drug abusers

- Haemophiliacs
- Infants born to infected mothers.

Health care workers: the risk to health care workers is low (estimated at around 0.4% in percutaneous injury with HIV-positive blood): exposure is mainly through needle-stick injuries in nursing, in surgery and in the laboratory. In addition there are rare instances, such as the well-publicized case of the Florida dentist who infected some of his patients, in which infection has been transmitted to patients through a medical procedure.

Geographical distribution: there are marked differences:

1. **Africa**: in sub-Saharan Africa, HIV infection – and AIDS – are epidemic: there is a high prevalence of HIV in sexually-active age groups (in some cities up to 20%). AIDS, and tuberculosis associated with it, are causing high mortality in many areas. Transmission is largely by heterosexual intercourse.

2. **Asia**: previously relatively free: AIDS is now endemic, and increasing at an alarming rate (mostly associated with prostitution) in Thailand and parts of India. Intravenous drug use is also an important factor in some areas.

3. **USA and Western Europe**: most infections have been acquired by homosexual anal intercourse between men: heterosexual spread is, as yet, responsible for only a minority of cases. Haemophiliac patients have been infected by contamination of factor VIII from infected donors (now controlled by blood screening and heat treatment). HIV infection is most prevalent in certain inner city populations. Drug abusers sharing needles also show a high prevalence of infection in some cities.

Virology

1. Retrovirus with genome structure as described above: the *env* gene, which codes for the main envelope glycoprotein and is involved in such immunity as is seen with this disease, shows considerable variation due to spontaneous mutation.

2. Electron microscopy: D-type retrovirus particle.

3. Grows in lymphocyte cultures, but with variable CPE. Co-cultivation with certain other cells results in syncytium formation and allows easier detection of virus growth.

Diagnosis

Serology: ELISA: if positive, confirm by additional ELISAs and western blot to analyse antibodies against individual virus proteins. HIV-1 and HIV-2 infections can be distinguished by serological tests as well as by PCR. The core (*gag*, P24) antigen is detectable at primary infection and in late disease.

Direct demonstration: *PCR*: for the detection of:

Virus RNA in blood and other body fluids.

Virus load: quantification of the amount of virus in blood can be important in monitoring the progress of the disease.

Infection in infants

Infection in infants is difficult to diagnose because of the persistence of maternal antibody in all babies born to infected mothers: HIV antibody persisting beyond 15 months is strong evidence of infection. PCR can detect infection at an early stage.

Treatment

Aimed at two targets:

1. HIV (see also Ch. 18): zidovudine (AZT): does not eradicate virus but improves survival: now recommended to be given in combination with didanosine (DDI) or zalcitabine (DDC): given to mothers during pregnancy reduces risk of transmission of virus to infants. Lamivudine, also an antiviral nucleoside, is now being used on a trial basis.

2. The associated opportunistic infections and tumours: treat with antimicrobial drugs and chemotherapy as appropriate.

18. Antiviral therapy

More drugs for treatment of viral infections are becoming available, and are now making a significant impact on disease. Table 18.1 shows the viruses for which effective therapy is available and the antiviral drugs with which they can be treated.

DRUGS ACTIVE AGAINST HERPESVIRUSES

Acyclovir

A breakthrough in antiviral therapy when introduced in 1982, because it is non-toxic to cells but strongly inhibits herpes simplex virus replication.

Viruses inhibited:

1. Herpes simplex virus types 1 and 2
2. Varicella-zoster – but less sensitive than herpes simplex virus.

Action: a nucleoside analogue that inhibits virus DNA synthesis: acyclovir is activated by phosphorylation by herpes-specific thymidine kinase, and is then inhibitory to the virus DNA polymerase. Varicella-zoster virus DNA polymerase is also sensitive – but less so – to this inhibition. Cellular DNA polymerase is resistant to the inhibition and, since the drug is

Table 18.1 Antiviral drugs

Viruses	Herpes simplex Varicella-zoster	Cytomegalovirus	Retrovirus HIV	Respiratory syncytial virus	Influenza A
Drugs	Acyclovir Valaciclovir Famciclovir	Ganciclovir Foscarnet	Zidovudine Didanosine Zalcitabine Lamivudine	Ribavirin*	Amantadine

*Also used for some other severe infections.

inactive unless in phosphorylated form, it is inactive in uninfected cells and therefore virtually non-toxic.

Latent virus is not eradicated, so that reactivations are not prevented – although they can be suppressed by long-term prophylaxis.

Used for treatment of:

1. herpes simplex: for example, encephalitis, genital herpes, cold sores, dendritic ulcer of the cornea, herpes simplex in the immunocompromised
2. varicella-zoster: severe varicella in leukaemic or other immunocompromised children; zoster: especially in the immunocompromised.

Note: acyclovir must be used in higher dosage for varicella- zoster than for herpes simplex.

Prophylactic use: prevents mucocutaneous reactivations of both herpes simplex and zoster in the immunocompromised (e.g. organ transplant recipients, leukaemia patients, etc.).

Administration: oral, topical (as a cream), intravenous (for severe infections).

Side-effects: minor: rashes, gastrointestinal disturbance, renal impairment – usually transient.

Valaciclovir

A prodrug of acyclovir, with better bio-availability: dosage is lower and less frequent than with acyclovir.

Indications: zoster and herpes simplex infections.

Administration: oral.

Famciclovir

Marketed for the treatment of zoster and genital herpes: the oral form of penciclovir: an agent similar in action to acyclovir, which is also activated by viral thymidine kinase in infected cells and which has good inhibitory activity against varicella-zoster virus.

Indications: zoster and genital herpes simplex.

Administration: oral.

Ganciclovir

A nucleoside analogue, active against cytomegalovirus.

Indications for use: severe, life-threatening cytomegalovirus infections in the immunocompromised, e.g. pneumonia, retinitis.

Administration: by slow intravenous infusion: orally for maintenance prophylaxis in transplant recipients.

Side-effects: neutropenia – and thrombocytopenia – are common: also fever, rash, impaired renal function and abnormal liver function tests.

Foscarnet

A pyrophosphate analogue which directly inhibits viral DNA polymerase and so viral replication: active against cytomegalovirus.

Indications for use: cytomegalovirus retinitis in AIDS patients.

Administration: by slow intravenous infusion.

Side-effects: renal toxicity, including acute renal failure; nausea, vomiting, malaise, hypocalcaemia, convulsions.

DRUGS ACTIVE AGAINST HIV

Most of those presently available are nucleoside analogues but, unlike acyclovir and related compounds, usually cause numerous and often severe side-effects. Most inhibit reverse transcriptase, and so viral replication. Resistant mutants emerge readily during the prolonged treatment necessary, and double or even triple therapy is now being recommended to prevent this.

Zidovudine (AZT)

Widely used, improves survival but does not eradicate the virus. Now recommended for use with either (or perhaps both) DDI or DDC (see below).

Administration: oral or by intravenous infusion.

Side-effects: anaemia, bone marrow depression with neutropenia; hepatic and renal impairment; nausea, vomiting, malaise.

Children: can be used for children.

Didanosine (DDI)

Used in combination with AZT or for patients in whom AZT is contraindicated or in whom there is deterioration while on AZT therapy.

Administration: oral.

Main side-effects: pancreatitis, peripheral neuropathy, raised uric acid in blood, diarrhoea.

Contraindications: breastfeeding; children (because safety in them is not yet established).

Zalcitabine (DDC)

Indications are where there is deterioration with AZT or for use in combination therapy.

Administration: oral.

Main side-effects: peripheral neuropathy, gastrointestinal symptoms, pancreatitis (but less often than with DDI), disturbance of liver function.

Contraindications: peripheral neuropathy, breastfeeding; children (in whom safety is not yet established).

Lamivudine

A nucleoside analogue that is showing some promise in early trials.

Protease inhibitors

Also showing some promise in trials: these inhibit by preventing cleavage of protein primary products – a necessary step in viral replication. They include ritonavir, indinavir and saquinavir (none of these yet licensed in early 1997).

DRUGS ACTIVE AGAINST OTHER VIRUSES

Ribavirin (tribavirin)

A nucleoside analogue active against a wide range of viruses, e.g. respiratory syncytial virus, arenaviruses, filoviruses.

Action: inhibits viral nucleic acid replication.

Indications for use: severe respiratory syncytial virus infection in infants, such as bronchiolitis, or bronchopneumonia; Lassa, Marburg and Ebola virus fevers.

Administration: for respiratory syncytial virus: by aerosol within a hood (which limits its usefulness); for other viruses: intravenously.

Side-effects: reticulocytosis; respiratory depression.

Amantadine

Active against influenza A but not influenza B. Effective for pro-phylaxis – and also for treatment if given early in infection: it has never been widely used, but might be useful in an influenza A pandemic if vaccine were not available.

Action: blocks penetration of virus into cells, probably with other antiviral activities also.

Indications for use: prevention and treatment of influenza A.

Administration: oral.

Side-effects: especially in the elderly: insomnia, nervousness, dizziness. Lower doses should be used in the elderly.

Interferon

Interferon alfa (see Ch. 1), prepared by recombinant technology or from stimulation of leucocyte cultures, has limited use against viruses.

Action: blocks virus transcription and protein synthesis.

Indications for use: chronic active hepatitis B, also used in chronic hepatitis C but long-term efficacy is not yet established. Used for certain haematological malignancies.

Administration: subcutaneous or intramuscular injection.

Side-effects: nausea, flu-like symptoms, tiredness, depression; sometimes, bone marrow depression.

19. Chlamydial diseases

Chlamydiae are widespread in human and animal populations. They are not viruses, but virus laboratories, by tradition, carry out diagnostic tests for them. This is because, despite the fact that they are really bacteria, they are unable to grow on inanimate media. Unlike viruses, they are sensitive to tetracycline and erythromycin.

There are three species of chlamydiae:

1. *Chlamydia trachomatis*
2. *Chlamydia pneumoniae*
3. *Chlamydia psittaci.*

Table 19.1 lists their serotypes and associated diseases.

Bacteriology of chlamydiae

1. Small, coccoid, Gram-negative bacteria.
2. Larger than most viruses: 250–500 nm: visible by light microscopy.

Table 19.1 Chlamydia

Species	Hosts	Main diseases	Serotypes
Chlamydia trachomatis	Humans	Oculogenital	D, E, F, G, H, I, J, K
		Trachoma	A, B, Ba, C
		Lymphogranuloma venereum	1, 2, 3
Chlamydia pneumoniae	Humans	Pneumonia	–
Chlamydia psittaci	Various animals (mainly birds)	Psittacosis	–

3. Grow – with difficulty – in cultures of McCoy or HeLa cells, with intracytoplasmic inclusions detected either by immunofluorescence (best with monoclonal antibody) or – less effective – by Giemsa staining: elementary bodies (produced during replication) are a characteristic feature of chlamydiae.
4. Grow in yolk sac of chick embryos.
5. Sensitive to antibiotics: tetracycline, erythromycin, sulphonamides.

CHLAMYDIA TRACHOMATIS

Causes a variety of clinical syndromes.

Non-gonococcal urethritis

Also known as *nonspecific urethritis*, and by far the commonest sexually-transmitted disease in Britain. Caused by *C. trachomatis* serotypes D to K.

Clinical features:

1. *Males*: acute urethritis with urethral discharge, frequency, dysuria: there may be cystitis, epididymitis and prostatitis – or proctitis in homosexual males. Reiter's syndrome (a triad of urethritis, arthritis and conjunctivitis) is seen in a low proportion (less than 1%) of cases.

2. *Females*: infection commonly involves the cervix. Usually symptomless, but sometimes accompanied by mild vaginitis with discharge. *C. trachomatis* causes salpingitis and pelvic inflammatory disease.

Treatment: tetracycline, erythromycin, azithromycin.

Ocular infection

C. trachomatis causes three types of eye infection:

1. Neonatal ophthalmia
2. Inclusion conjunctivitis
3. Trachoma.

Neonatal ophthalmia and inclusion conjunctivitis are due to the same serotypes as non-gonococcal urethritis (D to K): seen in countries with a temperate climate, such as Britain. Trachoma is a disease of tropical countries, and is due to different serotypes.

Neonatal ophthalmia

Caused by serotypes D to K and also called *inclusion blennorrhoea*. Seen in babies born to mothers with cervicitis, as a result of contamination acquired during passage through the infected birth canal.

Clinically: mucopurulent conjunctivitis, appearing 1–2 weeks after birth.

Treatment: oral erythromycin.

Inclusion conjunctivitis

A disease mainly of children but sometimes of adults also. Probably acquired by indirect contact from genital infection: outbreaks have been reported amongst children at swimming pools (*swimming pool conjunctivitis*). Caused by serotypes D to K.

Clinically: a follicular conjunctivitis with mucopurulent discharge: sometimes punctate keratitis if there is corneal involvement.

Treatment: oral tetracycline, erythromycin.

Trachoma

A major cause of blindness in the world and a scourge of tropical countries: tragically, a cause of needless suffering because it responds well to treatment: spread is from case to case by contact, contaminated fomites and flies. Caused by *C. trachomatis* serotypes A, B, Ba and C.

Clinically: a severe follicular conjunctivitis (Fig. 19.1) with pannus (i.e. invasion of the cornea by blood vessels): corneal scarring, which results in blindness, is a common sequela.

Treatment: topical or oral tetracycline, erythromycin, azithromycin.

Pneumonia

C. trachomatis (serotypes D to K) also causes pneumonia in neonates and in the immunocompromised.

Clinically: often preceded by upper respiratory symptoms: the pneumonia is relatively mild, with dry spasmodic cough and rapid breathing: the infants are not usually febrile. Chest X-rays show diffuse infiltration of the lungs.

Treatment: erythromycin.

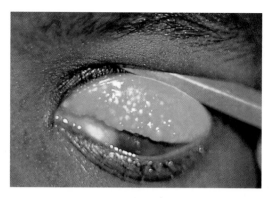

Fig. 19.1 Trachoma, showing severe follicular hyperplasia and papillary hyperplasia in the conjunctiva. (Photograph by the late Josef Sowa, reproduced, with the permission of the Stationery Office, from MRC Special Research Series Report No. 308.)

Lymphogranuloma venereum

A sexually transmitted disease, common in tropical countries, but almost unknown in temperate climates: if encountered in Britain the infection has usually been acquired abroad. Caused by *C. trachomatis* serotypes 1, 2 and 3.

Clinically:

1. *Males*: the primary lesion is a painless ulcer on the penis, which is often unnoticed. The disease then takes the form of the inguinal syndrome, in which there is painful enlargement of the inguinal and femoral lymph nodes, which later may suppurate to form buboes. Proctitis is a common complication in homosexual men.

2. *Females*: the genito-anorectal syndrome is the most common disease: infection involves the vagina and cervix – usually without symptoms – but the infection can then spread via the lymphatics to the rectum, causing proctitis with bleeding and purulent discharge from the anus.

Treatment: tetracycline, sulphonamides, erythromycin.

Diagnosis of *C. trachomatis* infections

Direct demonstration of antigen:
Specimens: swabs, smears from lesions.

Examine: by ELISA or by immunofluorescence for intracellular antigen, intracytoplasmic inclusions or elementary bodies – best with monoclonal antibody.

Isolation:

Specimens: genital or eye swabs.

Culture: in McCoy or HeLa cells.

Observe: for typical intracytoplasmic inclusions or elementary bodies, by immunofluorescence or Giemsa stain.

Note: in cases of suspected child abuse, it is essential to try and isolate chlamydiae.

Serology (less useful):

Immunofluorescence tests: type-specific, i.e. sera must be tested against the appropriate range of serotypes (i.e. D, E, F, G, H, I, J, K). Also used to detect the presence of IgM antibody, as an indicator of recent infection.

Complement fixation tests: genus-specific – i.e. only detect antibody to chlamydiae in general.

CHLAMYDIA PNEUMONIAE

Another species of human chlamydiae which causes respiratory infection is *C. pneumoniae* (formerly called TWAR, i.e. Taiwan acute respiratory agent).

Clinical features

Most infections are symptomless and reinfection appears to be common.

Respiratory: an 'atypical' mild pneumonia, sore throat with hoarseness, cough and fever: may be associated with asthma and wheezing, myocarditis and endocarditis.

A possible association with coronary artery disease is under investigation at present.

Epidemiology

Adults show a variable but quite high prevalence of antibody – around 20–70% – showing that infection is common in the community. Children under 5 years old rarely have antibody.

Outbreaks of pneumonia due to *C. pneumoniae* have been reported.

Diagnosis

Serology: immunofluorescence test.

Treatment

Tetracycline, erythromycin.

CHLAMYDIA PSITTACI

C. psittaci infects a variety of animals, but birds are the most important source of human disease. Infected birds often, but not always, show signs of disease – which is known as *ornithosis* in birds. In psittacine birds (e.g. budgerigars and parrots) the disease is also known as *psittacosis*. Most human cases are acquired from budgerigars or parrots, but other animals, e.g. sheep, may also be a source of infection.

In Britain, psittacosis is rare although the incidence has risen in recent years. Outbreaks of infection involving veterinary surgeons and workers in processing plants have been traced to infected flocks of ducks. Infection has been acquired from infected sheep during lambing, and may be severe in pregnant women.

Clinical features

Incubation period: 7–10 days.

Signs and symptoms: most often a primary atypical pneumonia: with fever, cough and dyspnoea, with extensive opacities in the lung fields on chest X-ray; headaches with CNS signs, including confusion, are common. Males are affected more often than females. Severity ranges from a mild influenza-like illness to a severe disease with generalized toxaemic features: rarely, infective endocarditis, as well as myocarditis and pericarditis: renal involvement and disseminated intravascular coagulation are occasional complications.

Mortality: sometimes fatal, although the case fatality rate is low (probably less than 1%).

Treatment: tetracycline, erythromycin.

Diagnosis

Serology: immunofluorescence tests; or complement fixation test: for rising titre against the chlamydial common group antigen: less sensitive, but still widely used in diagnosis.

20. Rickettsial diseases

Rickettsiae are not viruses, but are atypical bacteria: like chlamydiae, they are traditionally diagnosed in virus laboratories.

The most notorious rickettsial disease is typhus – an epidemic scourge in conditions of poverty and malnutrition (e.g. the German concentration camps of the Second World War) and of armies in the field. Typhus played a major part in the disintegration of Napoleon's army in the retreat from Moscow.

There are two genera within the family of rickettsiae:

- Rickettsia
- Coxiella.

The main difference between them is that coxiellae are resistant to drying.

RICKETTSIAE

Rickettsial diseases are transmitted by arthropod vectors, which are often also the reservoirs of the infection. Although not found in the UK, their distribution is world-wide. The main diseases are shown in Table 20.1.

Clinical features

Incubation period: 1–2 weeks.

Signs and symptoms: acute febrile illness with rash; malaise progressing to prostration; chills, myalgia, headache; haemorrhage and petechiae are common with the spotted fevers. Lymphadenopathy is seen in boutonneuse fever and scrub typhus.

Rash: a common, but not invariable, feature – usually maculopapular, except with rickettsialpox, in which the lesions are vesicular.

177

Table 20.1   Rickettsial diseases

Disease	Causal organism	Reservoir	Vector	Geographical distribution
Typhus group				
Typhus	*R. prowazekii*	Humans	Lice	Americas, Africa, Asia
Murine typhus	*R. typhi*	Rats, mice	Fleas	World-wide
Scrub typhus	*R. tsutsugamushi*	Mites	Mites	Far East
Spotted fever group				
Rocky Mountain spotted fever	*R. rickettsii*	Ticks	Ticks	Americas
Boutonneuse fever	*R. conorii*	Ticks	Ticks	Mediterranean, Africa
Queensland tick typhus	*R. australis*	Ticks	Ticks	Australia
North Asian tick fever	*R. sibirica*	Ticks	Ticks	Asian part of former Soviet Union, China, Mongolia
Rickettsialpox	*R. akari*	Mice	Mites	USA, former Soviet Union

Eschar: a skin ulcer, with blackened centre at the site of the infected bite, is a feature of boutonneuse fever and scrub typhus.

Recurrent infection is seen with typhus: *Brill-Zinsser disease*: recurrences may be years after the primary illness, and are usually mild.

Fatality: varies, but rickettsial diseases are often severe. Case fatality in untreated typhus is around 10–14% and in untreated Rocky Mountain spotted fever is 15–20%: other rickettsial diseases have lower mortality.

Epidemiology

Geographical distribution: rickettsial diseases exist as endemic foci in the areas listed in Table 20.1.

Transmission: via an infected vector, either by biting or by scratching faeces from infected vector into skin abrasions.

Epidemics: rare nowadays: the most important – at least historically – is typhus, classically a disease of war and famine.

Control of vectors is an effective method of cutting short an epidemic.

Bacteriology

1. Coccobacilli, approximately 300 nm in diameter
2. Visible by light microscopy
3. Replicate intracellularly by binary fission: best isolated in guinea-pigs, mice, or the yolk sac of chick embryos
4. Rapidly killed by drying
5. Sensitive to chloramphenicol and tetracycline.

Diagnosis

Serology: by immunofluorescence, ELISA test, sometimes complement fixation.
   Note: the older Weil-Felix reaction is no longer used.
   Isolation: rarely attempted, except for scrub typhus, in which the organism can be isolated by inoculation of patients' blood into mice.

Prophylaxis

A vaccine against typhus, containing the attenuated E strain of *R. prowazekii* has been developed.

Treatment

Tetracycline or chloramphenicol.

Q FEVER

Coxiella burnetii, the only member of the genus *Coxiella*, is the cause of Q (or 'query') fever. A sporadic disease in Britain, it was first described by Derrick in an outbreak of respiratory disease amongst meat workers in Queensland, Australia.

Clinical features

Incubation period: 2–3 weeks.
   Signs and symptoms: pyrexia of unknown origin (PUO); headache (a prominent symptom) with fever, generalized aches,

anorexia and slow pulse; some cases have enlargement of the liver with abnormal liver function tests; more rarely, splenomegaly. Q fever is a generalized septicaemic infection.

Pneumonia: about half the patients have the signs and symptoms of primary atypical pneumonia, with patchy consolidation of the lungs on chest X-rays.

Duration: about 2 weeks, but sometimes prolonged for 4 or more weeks, especially in patients over 40 years old.

Prognosis: is good and complete recovery is usual.

Infective endocarditis: rarely, Q fever is followed by chronic infection with involvement of the heart valves and formation of vegetations. The signs and symptoms are similar to those of bacterial infective endocarditis, i.e. fever, finger clubbing, anaemia, heart murmurs and splenomegaly; liver enlargement is common. The disease is usually – but not always – seen in patients with damaged heart valves: a much more serious disease than Q fever, and generally fatal if untreated.

Epidemiology

Animal reservoirs: sheep, cattle, other domestic animals and some wild animals; ticks are also infected and may play a role in spreading *C. burnetii* amongst animals, although generally transmission is via inhalation or ingestion of infected dust, straw, pasture, etc. At parturition, very large numbers of organisms are shed in the placenta, fluids and discharges, etc.

Geographical distribution: the disease is world-wide.

Route of human infection: mainly by inhalation of contaminated dust, placentas, fluids, etc. at parturition, sometimes by handling infected animals; infection can also be acquired by drinking unpasteurized, contaminated milk from infected cows, although this seems to be an unusual route.

Occupational hazard: animal workers have an increased risk of Q fever, but even in them the disease is rare.

Gender incidence: the majority of patients are male – probably reflecting the occupational hazard.

Seasonal incidence: Q fever is more common in spring and the early summer months.

Bacteriology

1. A typical rickettsia, but *C. burnetii* is resistant to drying

2. Grows in the yolk sac of chick embryos
3. Infects laboratory animals, e.g. guinea-pigs
4. Sensitive to tetracycline.

Diagnosis

Serology: complement fixation test: with two different preparations of *C. burnetii* as antigens:

Phase 1 antigen: freshly isolated strains of *C. burnetii* give no reaction with sera of acute cases, but react well with sera from patients with long-standing chronic infection (i.e. endocarditis).

Phase 2 antigen: strains of *C. burnetii*, after repeated passage in or adaptation to eggs, react well with sera of acute cases, as well as with sera from long-standing infections.

Acute Q fever

Serology: complement fixation test with phase 2 antigen.

Q fever endocarditis

Serology: complement fixation test with both phase 1 and phase 2 antigens: patients have high – usually very high – titres of antibodies to both antigens.

Isolation: by inoculation of guinea-pigs with material from valvular vegetations and spleen: after an interval the guinea-pig sera are tested for antibodies to *C. burnetii* by complement fixation test.

Direct demonstration: rarely done, but *C. burnetii* can be detected in smears of vegetations on heart valves (taken at operation for valve replacement), stained with Macchiavello's stain: *C. burnetii* is detected as minute red coccobacilli.

Treatment

Q fever can be successfully treated with tetracycline.

Endocarditis: requires long-term treatment with tetracycline; sometimes with rifampicin – this tends to suppress, rather than eradicate, the organism and careful follow-up is necessary. Removal of the diseased heart valves and replacement with valve prostheses has greatly improved the prognosis, and long-term survival can now be achieved.

21. Mycoplasma

There are two genera of mycoplasma that can cause human disease:

1. *Mycoplasma*
2. *Ureaplasma.*

Mycoplasma are bacteria which lack the peptidoglycan cell wall characteristic of bacteria: they can grow on bacteriological media.

The most important human pathogen in the group is *Mycoplasma pneumoniae*, which causes a disease originally known as 'virus pneumonia'; it is traditionally handled in virus laboratories.

MYCOPLASMA PNEUMONIAE

Clinical features

M. pneumoniae is primarily a respiratory pathogen. The infections it causes vary from mild pharyngitis to pneumonia.

Respiratory infections

1. **Primary atypical pneumonia**: formerly known as 'virus pneumonia', with symptoms of fever, hacking non-productive cough, often severe headache; marked weakness and tiredness are common. On chest X-ray there is patchy consolidation of the lungs, often more severe than the clinical features suggest: the disease lasts about 10 days, but sometimes symptoms persist for considerably longer.

2. **Other respiratory diseases**: *M. pneumoniae* also causes febrile bronchitis and tracheitis. Upper respiratory tract infections such as sinusitis, pharyngitis, coryza and otitis media (with bullous myringitis of the tympanic membrane) – and symptomless infection – are also common: most of these infections are probably not

recognized as due to mycoplasma, because not tested in the laboratory.

Note: primary atypical pneumonia is also caused – but more rarely – by *Coxiella burnetii* and *Chlamydia psittaci*.

Non-respiratory diseases

1. **Mucocutaneous eruptions**: *M. pneumoniae* also causes various types of rash – erythematous, maculopapular or vesicular. In some cases this is associated with conjunctival and mouth ulceration – the *Stevens-Johnson syndrome*.
2. **Neurological**: signs of CNS involvement are not uncommon in *M. pneumoniae* infection: most often meningism, aseptic meningitis or meningo-encephalitis, but cerebellar syndromes, transverse myelitis and nerve palsies have been reported.
3. **Haematological**: haemolytic anaemia sometimes complicates severe *M. pneumoniae* infection: probably due to the development of 'cold agglutinins' – a diagnostic feature of the disease (see below).

Epidemiology

M. pneumoniae infections are endemic in the community, but every 4 years there is an extensive epidemic (doubtless reflecting waning herd immunity after the previous outbreak).

Season: *M. pneumoniae* is a winter pathogen.

Age: most patients are children or young adults, but infection is commonly mild and asymptomatic in pre-school children.

Diagnosis

Serology: three tests are used:

1. *Complement fixation test* for demonstration of rising titre or – more often – stationary high titres (i.e. 256 or over).
2. *Immunofluorescence* to demonstrate specific IgM.
3. *Cold agglutinins*: patients commonly develop a haemagglutinin for human group O erythrocytes, which acts at 4°C. This interesting antibody seems to be produced as a result of antigenic sharing between *M. pneumoniae* and an antigen of human erythrocytes.

Treatment

Tetracycline; erythromycin in children.

OTHER MYCOPLASMA

Various *Mycoplasma* species inhabit human hosts as commensals:

- *M. hominis*: genital tract
- *M. orale*: mouth
- *M. salivarius*: mouth.
- *M. incognitus*: a variant of *M. fermentans*, has been separated as a cause of severe, multisystem failure in AIDS – but also in immunologically normal – patients.

M. orale and *M. salivarius* do not appear to be pathogenic. *M. hominis* can cause sepsis postpartum, post-abortion and in the neonate.

UREAPLASMA

Sometimes known as T (or tiny) strain mycoplasmas. *Ureaplasma urealyticum* is a commensal of the human genital tract. It is believed to cause some cases of non-gonococcal urethritis.

Recommended reading

Fields B N, Knipe D M, Howley P M (eds) 1996 Field's Virology, 3rd edn. Lippincott-Raven, Philadelphia

Mandell G L, Bennett J E, Dolin R 1995 Mandell, Douglas and Bennett's Principles and practice of infectious diseases, 4th edn. Churchill Livingstone, Edinburgh

Richman D D, Whitley R J, Hayden F G 1997 Clinical virology. Churchill Livingstone, New York

Zuckerman A J, Banatvala J E, Pattison J R (eds) 1994 Principles and practice of clinical virology, 3rd edn. Wiley, Chichester

Index

Acyclovir, 99, 102, 165
Adenoviruses, 50–53
    faecal, 51, 70–71, 72
Adsorption, 13
Adult T cell leukaemia/lymphoma,
        157
Aedes aegypti mosquito, 76
AIDS, 160–164
    see also HIV infection
    adenoviruses, 51
    cytomegalovirus retinitis, 105, 106,
        157
    foscarnet, 106, 167
    indicator infections, 161
    Kaposi's sarcoma, 109, 160
    paediatric, 161–162, 164
Alanine aminotransferase (ALT), 129
Alastrim, 125
Alphaviruses, 73, 78
Amantadine, 44, 169
Angiomatosis, bacillary, 160
Antibodies
    antibody response, 9–10
    neutralization, 10, 30–31, 35
    phagocytosis, 8–9
Antibody response, 9–10
Antibody-dependent cellular
        cytotoxicity (ADCC), 11
Antibody response, 9–10
Antigen-presenting cells, 10–11
Antigen tests, 31–32
Antigenic drift, 39, 41
Antigenic shift, 39, 41
Antigens, 9
    hepatitis B, 134
    Major Histocompatibility Complex,
        10–11
Antiviral therapy, 165–169
Aplastic crises, 120
Arboviruses, 73–80
Arenaviruses, 87–90

Arthralgia (painful joints)
    arboviruses, 77
    rubella, 116
Arthritis, 76, 77
Arthropods, 73–80
Aspirin, 38, 57
Astroviruses, 71
Automated technology, 27
Azithromycin, 172, 173

B lymphocytes, 9, 10
Baltimore classification, 15
Bell's palsy, 102
BK virus, 141–142
Blennorrhoea, inclusion (neonatal
        ophthalmia), 172, 173
Bone marrow transplantation, 51, 106
Bornholm disease (pleurodynia;
        epidemic myalgia), 60, 62
Boutonneuse fever, 177, 178
Bovine spongiform encephalopathy,
        145, 147–148
Brill-Zinsser disease, 178
Bronchiolitis, 46, 47, 112
Bronchitis, 112, 183
Bronchopneumonia, 112
Bunyaviruses, 73, 77, 79, 90
Burkitt's lymphoma, 108
Butcher's warts, 150–151

Caliciviruses, 71–72
California encephalitis, 73
Candidiasis, 160
Capsid, 2
Capsomeres, 2
Cataract, 117
CD4 positive helper T cells, 10–11
CD8 positive cytotoxic T cells, 10–11
Cell death, 3
Cell-mediated immunity, 10–11
Central European encephalitis, 74–75

Central nervous system
  see Neurological diseases
Cervical cancer, 151
Cervical dysplasia, 160
Cervical intraepithelial neoplasia
  (CIN), 151, 160
Chemotaxis, 9
Chick embryo culture, 3, 35
Chickenpox (varicella), 100–101
Chikungunya, 77
Chlamydia pneumoniae, 175–176
Chlamydia psittaci, 176
Chlamydia trachomatis, 172–175
Chlamydial diseases, 171–176
Chloramphenicol, 179
Chlorine, 7
Chloroform, 7
Choriomengitis, lymphocytic, 89–90
Cirrhosis, 132, 136
Cold agglutinins, 184
Cold effects, 6
Cold sores, 96–97
Common cold, 46, 47, 53
Competitive assay, 28
Complement, 8–9
Complement fixation test, 30
Condylomata acuminata, 149
Conjunctiva, 8
Conjunctivitis
  acute haemorrhagic, 60, 62
  adenoviruses, 50
  enteroviruses, 60, 62
  inclusion, 172, 173
  primary herpes simplex, 94
  swimming pool, 173
Cornea
  dendritic ulcer, 97
  pannus, 173
  transplant, 83
Coronaviruses, 53
Coxiella burnetii, 179–181
Coxsackieviruses, 53, 59, 62, 63
Creutzfeldt-Jakob disease (CJD), 56,
  144–145
  new variant (vCJD), 144, 148
Crimean-Congo haemorrhagic fever,
  77
Croup (acute
  laryngotracheobronchitis), 46,
  112
Cystitis, 172
  acute haemorrhagic, 51
Cytokines, 9, 11–12
Cytomegalovirus, 57, 103–106
  congenital disease, 104
  postnatal, 104–105

Cytopathic effect (CPE), 3, 7–8, 34
Cytotoxic T cells, 10–11

Dane particles, 133–134
Deafness
  congential cytomegalovirus infection,
    104
  mumps, 115
  rubella, 117
Defence mechanisms
  non-specific, 8–9
  specific (immunological), 9–12
Dehydration, 67
Delta agent (hepatitis D), 137–138
Dementia, AIDS, 56
Dendritic cells, 11
Dendritic ulcer, 97
Dengue, 76–77
Dengue haemorrhagic shock syndrome,
  77
Dermatitis, contagious pustular (orf),
  125
Dermatomes, 101
Diarrhoea, 53, 67–72
Didanosine (DDI), 164, 167–168
Direct early antigen fluorescent foci
    test (DEAFF), 105
Direct tests, 31–33
Disinfectants, 7
DNA-dependent DNA polymerase, 16,
  17
DNA viruses
  classification, 4
  double-stranded, 15–18
  replication, 15–19
Dorsal root ganglia, 101
Drug abusers, 131, 137, 138, 139,
    158–159, 162, 163
Drying effects, 7

Early proteins, 17
Eastern equine encephalitis, 73, 74, 75
Ebola virus disease, 86–87
Echoviruses, 53, 59, 62, 63
Electron microscopy, 33, 35
Encephalitis, 55
  acute necrotizing, 95
  arbovirus, 73–75
  herpes, 95, 99
  measles, 112–113
  post-infectious, 56, 113, 116
  primary, 56
Encephalopathies
  AIDS, 56
  bovine spongiform, 145, 147–148
  spongiform, 142–144
  transmissible mink, 147

Endocarditis, 180, 181
Enteroviruses, 53, 59–65, 72
Entry, virus, 13
Envelope, 2
Enzyme-linked immunosorbent assay (ELISA), 27, 28–29, 31–32
Epidermodysplasia verruciformis, 149
Epididymitis, 172
Epstein-Barr virus, 57, 106–109
Erythema infectiosum (slapped cheek disease; fifth disease), 111, 120–121
Erythromycin, 171, 172, 173, 174, 176, 185
Eschar, 178
Ether, 7
Exanthema subitum (roseola infantum), 109

Facial nerve palsy, 101
Factor VIII, 130, 132, 136, 163
Fallot's tetralogy, 117
Famciclovir, 99, 103, 136, 166
Far Eastern encephalitis, 75
Fastidious viruses, 51, 70
Fatal familial insomnia, 144
Febrile illness
    arboviruses, 75–78
    enteroviruses, 60, 61
    lymphocytic choriomeningitis, 90
Fibrosarcomata, 156
Fifth disease (erythema infectiosum), 111, 120–121
Filoviruses, 87
Flaviviruses, 73, 79
Fluorescein dye, 29, 32
Formaldehyde, 7
Foscarnet, 106, 167

Ganciclovir, 106
Gastroenteritis, viral, 51, 67–72
Gastrointestinal tract defence mechanism, 8
Genital herpes, 95, 96, 97, 99
Genital warts, 149, 151
Genito-anorectal syndrome, 174
Genome, 1–2
Gerstmann-Straussler-Scheinker disease, 144
Giant cell pneumonia, 46, 112
Gingivostomatitis, 94
Glandular fever see Infectious mononucleosis
Glutaraldehyde, 7
Guanarito virus, 89
Guillain-Barré syndrome, 43, 57

Haemadsorption, 4, 34–35
Haemagglutination-inhibition, 30, 40
Haemagglutination test, 35
Haemagglutinin, 4, 40, 41
Haemophiliacs, 130, 132, 137, 139, 163
Haemophilus influenzae infection, 38
Haemorrhagic fever with renal syndrome, 90
Haemorrhagic fevers
    arboviruses, 75–78
    Crimean Congo, 77
    non-arthropod-borne, 86–91
    South American, 89
Hairy leukoplakia, 160
Hand, foot and mouth disease, 60, 62
Hantaan virus, 90
Hantavirus pulmonary syndrome, 90
Hantaviruses, 90–91
Healthcare workers, 163
Heat effects, 6
Helper T cells, 9, 10–11
Hepatitis
    anicteric, 129
    chronic, 129
    chronic active, 132
    chronic persistent, 132
    cytomegalovirus, 104–105
    fulminant with massive liver necrosis (acute yellow atrophy), 129
    herpes, 95
    yellow fever, 76
Hepatitis A, 129–131
    complications, 129
    vaccine, 130–131
Hepatitis B, 131–136
    antigenic structure, 134
    carriers, 131
    complications, 129
    hepatitis D, 137–138
    replication, 19
    treatment, 136
    vaccine, 135
    viral, 127–139
Hepatitis C (non-A-non-B hepatitis), 136–137
    complications, 129
Hepatitis D (delta agent), 138
Hepatitis E, 138–139
    complications, 129
Hepatitis F, 139
Hepatitis G, 139
Hepatitis, viral, 127–139
Hepatosplenomegaly, 117
Herpangina, 60, 62

Herpes simplex virus, 93–99
  antiviral therapy, 165–166
Herpesviruses, 93–109
  antiviral therapy, 165–167
Histiocytes, 8
HIV infection, 159
  see also AIDS
  clinical features, 159–160
  dementia/encephalopathy, 56
  treatment, 161, 164, 167–168
  viral replication, 23
Host response, 8–12
HTLV-I, 157–158
HTLV-II, 158–159
Human diploid cell vaccine (HDCV), 85
Human herpes virus-6 (HHV-6), 109
Human herpes virus-7 (HHV-7), 109
Human herpes virus-8 (HHV-8), 109
Human immunodeficiency virus see
  AIDS; HIV infection
Humoral (antibody) response, 9–10
Hydrogen peroxide, 7
Hydrophobia, 81
Hydrops fetalis, 120–121
Hypochlorite solution, 7
Hyponatraemia, 67, 68

IgA, 10
IgG, 10, 11
  detection, 31
IgM, 9
  detection, 31
Immunocompromised patients
  see also Transplant patients
  adenoviruses, 51
  BK virus, 142
  cytomegalovirus infection, 105
  Epstein-Barr virus, 107
  erythema infectiosum, 121
  ganciclovir, 106
  human herpes virus-6, 109
  parainfluenza viruses, 46
  warts, 151
Immunofluorescence, 29, 32, 35
Immunoglobulins, 9–10
Immunological response, 9–12
Immunosuppressive therapy see
  Transplant patients
Inclusion bodies, 33
Indinavir, 168
  host response, 8–12
  laboratory diagnosis, 27–36
  latent, 3
  persistent, 52

Infectious mononucleosis
  cytomegalovirus, 105
  Epstein-Barr virus, 107–108
Infectivity, 15
Influenza virus, 37–43
  antigenic structure, 40
  clinical features, 37–38
  diagnosis, 42–43
  epidemics, 37, 38–39, 41–42
  epidemiology, 38–39
  haemagglutination, 40
  influenza A, 38, 40–42, 57, 169
  influenza B, 38, 42, 57
  influenza C, 38
  replication, 23
  vaccination, 43, 57
  virology, 39–40
  virus types, 38
Inguinal syndrome, 174
Inoculation, 7, 34
Insomnia, fatal familial, 144
Interferon-alpha, 136, 137, 169
Interferons, 11–12
Interleukins, 11
Intussusception, 51
Iodine, 7

Japanese encephalitis, 74, 75
  vaccine, 80
Jaundice, 127–129
JC virus, 141–142
Joint pain see Arthralgia
Junin virus, 89

Kaposi's sarcoma, 109, 160
Kaposi's varicelliform eruption, 95
Keratitis
  chlamydial, 173
  herpes simplex, 94, 97
Keratoconjunctivitis, epidemic, 51
Killer (K) cells, 11
Koplik's spots, 111
Kupffer cells, 8
Kuru, 145–146

Laboratory animals, 3, 36
Lamivudine, 136, 164, 168
Laryngeal papilloma, 149, 151
Laryngotracheobronchitis, acute
  (croup), 46, 112
Lassa fever, 8–89
Late proteins, 18
Leukaemia viruses, 156–157
Listeriosis, 160
Liver cancer, 129, 133, 136

Louping ill, 73
Lymphocytic choriomeningitis, 89–90
Lymphogranuloma venereum, 174
Lymphokine-activated killer (LAK)
    cells, 11
Lymphoma, 57
    Burkitt's, 108
Lymphoproliferative disease, 107
Lysis, 10–11
Lyssaviruses, 83

Machupo virus, 89
Macrophages, 8–9, 11
Major Histocompatibility Complex
    (MHC) antigens, 10–11
Malaria, 108
Marburg disease, 86–87
Measles, 111–114
Meningitis, aseptic, 55, 56, 60–61
    epidemics, 63
    lymphocytic choriomeningitis, 90
    mumps, 114–115
    Mycoplasma pneumoniae, 184
Meningoencephalitis
    lymphocytic choriomeningitis, 90
    mumps, 114, 120
    Mycoplasma pneumoniae, 184
Mesenteric adenitis, 51
Microcephaly, 104
Microglia, 8
Molluscum contagiosum, 124, 125
Monkeypox, 125
Mononucleosis
    with cervical lymphadenopathy, 109
    infectious *see* Infectious
        mononucleosis
mRNA, 13–14
    early/late, 16
Mumps, 114–116
    meningoencephalitis, 120
Murray Valley encephalitis, 74
Myalgia, epidemic (Bornholm disease),
    60, 62
Mycoplasma, 183–185
Mycoplasma fermentans, 185
Mycoplasma hominis, 185
Mycoplasma incognitus, 185
Mycoplasma orale, 185
Mycoplasma pneumoniae, 183–185
Mycoplasma salivarius, 185
Myocarditis, 60, 62
Myositis, 64
Myringitis, bullous, 183

Nasopharyngeal carcinoma, 108

Natural killer (NK) cells, 11
Negri bodies, 82, 84
Neonates
    cytomegalovirus infection, 104
    herpes infection, 95
    ophthalmia (inclusion
        blennorrhoea), 172, 173
    varicella, 100, 103
Nephropathia epidemica, 90
Neuralgia, post-zoster, 102
Neuraminidase, 40
Neurological diseases, 55–57
    acute, 55
    chronic, 55–57, 141–148
    enteroviruses, 60–61
Neutralization, 10, 30–31, 35
Neutropenia, 106
Neutrophil polymorphonuclear
    leucocytes, 8
Non-antibody-dependent cytotoxicity,
    11
Nucleic acid genome, 1–2

O'nyong-nyong, 77
Oncogenes
    adenoviruses, 52
    Epstein-Barr virus, 107
    retroviruses, 154–155
Oophoritis, 115
Ophthalmia, neonatal (inclusion
        blennorrhoea), 172, 173
Ophthalmic nerve, 101
Opsonization, 8
Orchitis, 115
Orf (contagious pustular dermatitis),
    125
Ornithosis, 176
Orthomyxoviruses, 39
Otitis media, 112
Otitis media, 183
Otitis media, 49
Oxidizing agents, 7

Pancreatitis, 115
Papillomaviruses
    cancer, 151–152
    warts, 149–152
Parainfluenza viruses, 45–47
    replication, 21–23
Paralysis
    arboviruses, 74, 75
    coxsackievirus, 64
    poliovirus *see* Poliomyelitis
    rabies, 81
Paravaccinia (pseudocowpox), 125

Parotitis, 114–115, 162
Parotitis, 162
  human parvovirus B19, 120–121
  replication, 19
Patent ductus arteriosus, 117
Paul-Bunnell test, 108
Pelvic inflammatory disease, 160, 172
Penciclovir, 166
Pericarditis, 60, 62
Peripheral neuropathy, 160
Phagocytosis, 8–9
Pharyngitis, 50, 116, 183
Phenols, 7
Plantar warts, 149, 151
Plasma cells, 9
Pleurodynia (Bornholm disease), 60, 62
Pneumococcal infection, 38
Pneumonia
  Chalmydia pneumoniae, 175
  Chlamydia psittaci, 176
  Chlamydia trachomatis, 173
  cytomegalovirus, 105
  giant cell, 46, 112
  lymphoid interstitial, 162
  parainfluenza virus, 46
  primary influenzal, 37–38
  Q fever, 180
  respiratory syncytial virus, 47
  secondary bacterial, 38
  varicella, 100
  virus pneumonia (*Mycoplasma pneumoniae*), 183
Poliomyelitis, 55, 60, 61
  epidemic, 63
  vaccine, 61, 63, 64–65
Polioviruses, 59
  epidemic aseptic meningitis, 63
  eradication, 65
  paralysis *see* Poliomyelitis
  replication, 20
  vaccination, 61, 63, 64–65
Polyarthritis, 76, 77
Polymerase chain reaction (PCR), 32
Polymorphonuclear leucocytes, 11
Polyomaviruses, 141
Poxviruses, 123–125
Pregnancy
  cytomegalovirus infection, 103
  hepatitis B, 132
  hepatitis E, 138
  human polyomaviruses, 142
  rubella, 116
  varicella, 100
Primary hepatocellular carcinoma, 129, 133, 136

Prions, 141, 143–144
Probes, 32
Proctitis, 172, 174
Progressive multifocal leucoencephalopathy, 56, 141–142
β-Propiolactone, 7
Prostatitis, 172
Protease inhibitors, 168
Provirus 23, 25
Proviruses, 19
Pseudocowpox, 125
Psittacosis, 176
Pulmonary artery stenosis, 117
Purpura, thrombocytopaenic, 116, 117, 160
Purtillo's syndrome, 107
Puumala virus, 90

Q fever, 179–181
Quarantine, 82–83

Rabies, 81–86
Radial haemolysis, 30
Radioimmunoassay (RIA), 29
Ramsay Hunt's syndrome, 101–102
Rashes
  enteroviruses, 62
  measles, 111
  Mycoplasma pneumoniae, 184
  parvovirus B19, 120
  rickettsial, 177
  rubella, 116
Reducing agents, 7
Reiter's syndrome, 172
Renal dialysis units, 132
Reoviruses, 23
Respiratory syncytial virus, 47–49
Respiratory tract, 8
Respiratory tract infections, 45–53
  influenza *see* Influenza virus
  measles, 112
  rotaviruses, 69
Retinitis, cytomegalovirus, 105, 106, 167
Retroviruses, 153–164
  animal, 153–157
  endogenous, 156
  human, 157–164
  replication, 19, 23–25
Reverse transcriptase, 24, 154
Reye's syndrome, 38, 57
Rhinoviruses, 49–50
Ribavirin (tribavirin), 49, 89, 91, 168
Rickettsiae, 177–179
Rickettsial diseases, 177–181

Rickettsialpox, 177
Rifampicin, 181
Rift Valley fever, 77–78
Ritonavir, 168
RNA-dependent RNA polymerase, 20, 21, 23
RNA viruses
    classification, 4–5
    double-stranded segmented, 19, 23
    influenza, 39
    replication, 19–25
    single-strand negative-sense (minus-sense), 19, 21–23
    single-strand positive-sense (plus-sense), 19, 20–21
Rocio virus, 73
Rocky Mountain spotted fever, 178
Roseola infantum, 109
Ross River virus, 77
Rotaviruses, 69–70
Rubella, 116–119
    congenital infection, 116–118
    vaccine, 118
Rubella syndrome, 117–118

Sabia virus, 89
Sabin vaccine, 64–65
St Louis encephalitis, 73, 75
Salk vaccine, 65
Salpingitis, 172
Saquinavir, 168
Sarcoma viruses, 156
Scrapie, 146
Scrub typhus, 177, 178, 179
Seoul virus, 91
Serology, 27–31
Shingles (zoster), 101–103, 160
Sickle cell anaemia, 120
Sin nombre virus, 90
Single radial haemolysis, 30
Sinusitis, 49, 183
Skin, 8
    cancer, 151
Slapped cheek disease (erythema infectiosum), 111, 120–121
Slow virus diseases, 141
Small round structured viruses (SRSVs), 71–72
Smallpox (variola), 123, 125
Soluble (S) antigen, 40
South American haemorrhagic fevers, 89
Spherocytosis, hereditary, 120
Spongiform encephalopathies, 142–144
Squamous cell carcinoma, 149, 151

Staphylococcus aureus infection, 38
Stevens-Johnson syndrome, 184
Subacute sclerosing panencephalitis, 56, 112–113, 118
Sulphonamides, 174

T lymphocytes, 9, 10–11
Tacaribe complex, 89
Tanapox, 125
Tetracycline, 171, 172, 173, 174, 176, 179, 181, 185
Thalassaemia, 120
Thrombocytopaenic purpura, 116, 117, 160
Thymidine kinase, 17
Thyroiditis, 115
Tick-borne encephalitis, 74, 75
    vaccine, 80
Tissue culture, 3, 33–35
Toroviruses, 53, 72
Tracheitis, 183
Trachoma, 172, 173
Transaminases, 129
Transcription, 13–14
Transformation, 3
Transplant patients
    adenoviruses, 51
    bone marrow transplantation, 51, 106
    corneal transplant, 83
    cytomegalovirus infection, 103, 105
    herpes simplex virus infection, 97
    human herpes virus-6, 109
    human polyomaviruses, 142
    varicella-zoster immunoglobulin, 103
Tribavirin (ribavirin), 89, 91, 168
Trigeminal ganglion, 95–96, 101
Tropical spastic paraparesis, 56, 157, 158
Tumour necrosis factor, 11
Typhus, 177, 178
    vaccine, 179

Ultraviolet irradiation, 7
Uncoating, 13
Ureaplasma urealyticum, 185
Urethritis, non-gonococcal (nonspecific), 172, 185
Urinary tract, 8
Uveitis, 97

Vaccination
    dengue, 79
    eastern equine encephalitis, 79
    hepatitis A, 130–131
    hepatitis B, 135

Vaccination (*contd*)
  influenza, 43, 57
  Japanese encephalitis, 80
  measles, 112
  measles, mumps and rubella
      (MMR), 111, 112, 115, 118,
      119–120
  poliomyelitis, 61, 63, 64–65
  rabies, 82, 85–86
  respiratory syncytial virus, 47–48
  rubella, 111, 118
  smallpox, 123, 125
  tick-borne encephalitis, 80
  varicella-zoster, 103
  western equine encephalitis, 79
  wild animals, 83, 86
  yellow fever, 79–80
Vaccinia virus, 125
Valaciclovir, 99, 166
Varicella (chickenpox), 57, 100–101
Varicella-zoster virus, 100–103
  antiviral therapy, 165–166
  immunoglobulin (ZIG), 103
Variola (smallpox), 123, 125
Venezuelan equine encephalitis, 74,
      75
Ventricular septal defect, 117
Viraemia, 60, 61
  hepatitis A, 129, 130
  hepatitis B, 131
Virion, 2
Viruses
  assembly, 14, 18
  Baltimore classification, 15
  biochemistry, 15–25
  classification, 4
  cultivation, 2–3
  detection, 27–33
  diseases, 7–8

effects on cells, 3–4
genomes, 14–15
growth cycle, 13–14
growth detection, 34–35
identification, 35
infection *see* Infection
infectivity, 15
invasiveness, 7–8
isolation, 33–36
large, 15
nucleic acid genomes, 14–15
nucleic acid synthesis, 14
physical/chemical agent effects, 6–7
properties, 1
properties, 15
protein synthesis, 14, 17–18
release, 14
replication, 13–25
small, 15
structure, 1–2
symmetry, 2
transcription, 13–14

Warts, 149–152
  butcher's, 150–151
  genital, 149, 151
  plantar, 149, 151
Western blot, 28–29
Western equine encephalitis, 73, 75
  vaccine, 79
Whitlow, 94

Yellow fever, 76
  vaccine, 79–80

Zalcitabine (DDC), 164, 168
Zidovudine (AZT), 161, 164, 167
Zoonoses, 81–91
Zoster (shingles), 101–103, 160